GOOD FORMULAS

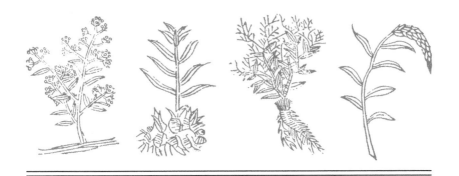

GOOD FORMULAS

EMPIRICAL EVIDENCE IN MID-IMPERIAL
CHINESE MEDICAL TEXTS   *Ruth Yun-ju Chen*

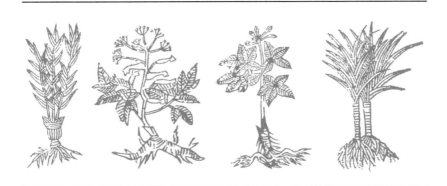

University of Washington Press / *Seattle*

Good Formulas was made possible in part by a grant from the Traditional Chinese Culture and Society Book Fund, established through generous gifts from Patricia Buckley Ebrey and Thomas Ebrey.

This publication was also supported by grants from the Association for Asian Studies First Book Subvention Program and the Chiang Ching-kuo Foundation for International Scholarly Exchange.

Copyright © 2023 by the University of Washington Press
Design by Mindy Basinger Hill
Composed in 10.2/14pt Minion Pro

All rights reserved. No part of this publication may be reproduced or transmitted in any form or by any means, electronic or mechanical, including photocopy, recording, or any information storage or retrieval system, without permission in writing from the publisher.

UNIVERSITY OF WASHINGTON PRESS *uwapress.uw.edu*

LIBRARY OF CONGRESS CATALOGING-IN-PUBLICATION DATA

Names: Chen, Yunru (Researcher in Chinese history), author.
Title: Good formulas : empirical evidence in mid-imperial Chinese
    medical texts / Ruth Yun-Ju Chen.
Description: Seattle : University of Washington Press, [2023] | Includes
    bibliographical references and index.
Identifiers: LCCN 2022062236 | ISBN 9780295751382 (hardback) |
    ISBN 9780295751399 (paperback) | ISBN 9780295751405 (ebook)
Subjects: LCSH: Medicine, Chinese—History—To 1500. | Medical
    literature—China—History—To 1500.
Classification: LCC R601 .C442 2023 | DDC 610.951—dc23/eng/20230228
LC record available at https://lccn.loc.gov/2022062236

⊗ This paper meets the requirements of ANSI/NISO Z39.48-1992
    (Permanence of Paper).

To my family and my teachers

Contents

Acknowledgments *ix*

Chinese Historical Dynasties *xi*

Introduction *1*

ONE New Criteria for "Good" Medical Formulas *14*

TWO Textual Claims and Local Investigations *44*

THREE Demonstration of Medical Virtuosity *76*

FOUR The Search for Therapies in the Far South *104*

Conclusion *132*

Glossary of Chinese Characters *145*

Notes *153*

Bibliography *181*

Index *203*

Acknowledgments

OVER THE PAST DECADE, while writing this book, I have benefited enormously from the help and support of many colleagues and contributors. In the early stages of the project, Elisabeth Hsu contributed her expertise on the history of medicine in early China and medical anthropology, Hilde De Weerdt contributed her knowledge of the history of middle-period China, and Marta Hanson shared comparative insights into the history of medicine in early modern China and Europe.

For the time they devoted to reading and commenting on draft chapters and related materials, I owe thanks to the following people: Robert Chard, Barend Ter Haar, Peter Ditmanson, Erica Charters, Chen Hsiu-Fen, TJ Hinrichs, Benjamin Elman, Cheng Hsiao-wen, Liu Yan, Margaret Ng, Michael Stanley Baker, Dolly Yang, Wu Hsiao-chun, Lin Hsin-yi, Chen Shaiu-yun, Chen Hao, Stephen Boyanton, Tung Yung-chang, Tsui Lik Hang, Liu Qian, Marshall Crag, Samuel Yin, and Guo Ting. I also appreciate the many valuable suggestions that two anonymous reviewers contributed.

Over the past several years, I have presented portions of the manuscript at various conferences and institutions, including but not limited to the Association for Asian Studies Annual Conference, the first and second Conferences on Middle Period China, the Conference on Tang-Song Transitions, the National Palace Museum, the National Central Library, and the Institute of History and Philology at Academia Sinica. I appreciate the many useful comments I was fortunate to receive from the hosts of and audiences at these conferences and lectures.

Since 2015, Academia Sinica has provided me with an ideal scholarly home, and I thank its members, particularly Huang Kuan-chung, Sean Hsiang-lin Lei,

Chu Ping-yi, Li Shang-jen, Kevin Chang, Tai Li-chuan, Chen Wen-yi, Cheng Ya-ju, Liu Hsin-ning, Albert Wu, Li Ren-yuan, Lee Chang-yuan, Lee Hsiu-ping, and Chang Che-chia. The extraordinary mentorship and friendship that Lee Jen-der offered has helped me navigate through my early career.

While I was writing this book, I was fortunate to encounter many sharp and inspiring minds who supported me professionally and personally at various stages of this project: Charles Hartman, Shigehisa Kuriyama, Angela Ki Che Leung, Bian He, Zuo Ya, Hilary Smith, John Moffett, James Flowers, Duan Xiaolin, Yu Xinzhong, Chang Chia-feng, Chen Yuan-peng, Fang Cheng-hua, Liao Hsien-huei, Chang Wei-ling, Debby Chih-yen Huang, Hsu Kai-hsiang, Elisabeth Forster, Yegor Grebnev, Rens Krijgsman, Yuan Ai, Dongsob Ahn, Hung Kuang-chi, Wang Hsien-chun, Wu Hsin-fang, Chen Kuan-fei, Tsai Tian-i, Tu Hsuan-ying, Liu Shih-hsun, Wang Fei-hsien, Hsia Ke-chin, and many others.

Editors and staff members at the University of Washington Press (UWP), with their professional help, assured that the production and publication of this book proceeded smoothly. I especially thank Lorri Hagman, Marcella Landri, Beth Fuget, Joeth Zucco, David Schlangen, Richard Isaac (copyediting), Susan Stone (indexing), and Megan Michel Mendonça (proofreading). I also thank William Barnett, whose copyediting helped me refine the language. All remaining errors, of course, are mine.

In addition, I thank the National Central Library, the Institute of History and Philology, and the Library of Congress for granting permission to use their images in the book. Preparation and publication of this book was generously supported by grants from Taiwan's National Science and Technology Council (110-2410-H-001-004). I thank the Center for Chinese Studies in Taiwan for permission to include portions of my article "Accounts of Treating Zhang ('miasma') Disorders in Song-Dynasty Lingnan: Remarks on Changing Literary Forms of Writing Experience" (*Hanxue yanjiu* [Chinese Studies] 34, no. 3 [September 2016]: 205–54) in chapter 4.

Finally, the everlasting love and support of my parents, Chen Kuen-ning and Liang Ching-kang, and my grandmother, Yang Hsiang-mei, have sustained me over these years and bestowed on me the courage to proceed. My husband Li-kung's words and company have provided constant encouragement. I am highly blessed to have benefited from the help of so many during my intellectual journey. I could not have written this book without it.

Chinese Historical Dynasties

Shang (ca. 1600–1046 BCE)
Zhou (ca. 1046–256 BCE)
   Western Zhou (ca. 1046–771 BCE)
   Eastern Zhou (770–256 BCE)
      Spring and Autumn Period (770–476 BCE)
      Warring States Period (476–221 BCE)
Qin (221–206 BCE)
Han (202 BCE–220 CE)
   Western Han (202 BCE–8 CE)
   Xin (9–23)
   Eastern Han (25–220)
Era of Division (220–589)
   Three Kingdoms (220–280)
   Jin (266–420)
   Sixteen Kingdoms (304–439)
   Northern Dynasties (386–581)
      Northern Wei (386–534)
      Eastern Wei (534–550)
      Western Wei (535–557)
      Northern Qi (550–577)
      Northern Zhou (557–581)
   Southern Dynasties (420–589)
      Liu-Song (420–479)
      Southern Qi (479–502)
      Liang (502–557)
      Chen (557–589)

Sui (581–619)
Tang (618–907)
Five Dynasties and Ten Kingdoms (907–960)
Liao (Khitan) (907–1125)
Song (960–1279)
　　Northern Song (960–1127)
　　Southern Song (1127–1279)
Jin (Jurchen) (1115–1234)
Yuan (Mongol) (1271–1368)
Ming (1368–1644)
Qing (Manchu) (1636–1911)

GOOD FORMULAS

Introduction

DURING THE SONG DYNASTY (960–1279), China experienced a flood of information. With this publishing boom, which created a new learning environment for medicine, a strategy for narrating empirical evidence and for substantiating knowledge claims gained salience in medical literature. We see one example of this strategy in Shen Kuo (1031–1095), a high-ranking civil official, who purportedly once brought a sick person back to life, even though he had never received expert medical training.[1] Shen wrote that, while riding in a boat, he saw a boatman's son who was so ill that he had lost consciousness and was seemingly on his last breath. Although Shen was not confident that he could treat the young man effectively, he did not have the heart to leave him to die. Shen hence generously shared his own pills with the suffering man—Rose-Storax Pills (Suhexiang Wan), medicines made using expensive and luxurious aromatics, such as agarwood and musk. After being administered four of the pills, the man regained consciousness and then recovered. Shen Kuo narrated this healing event in a medical treatise that he completed late in life, *Good [Medical] Formulas* (Liangfang). In *Good Formulas*, Shen appended a narrative of this healing event to the medical formula for the Rose-Storax Pill, which he included in the treatise as proof of its miraculous therapeutic efficacy.[2] This case narrative, which illustrated Shen's generosity to a dying stranger, additionally demonstrated his benevolence. *Good Formulas* soon circulated across Song China, and other Song authors often cited this treatise.

In the Song era, narratives based on authors' personal experience (such as the abovementioned healing event) proliferated across medical literature as a strategy for enhancing the credibility and trustworthiness of a given treatise. Personal experience in the narratives encompassed authors' medical cases, their encounters with the sick, their witness of and oral inquiry into others' hands-on experience, and their observations of local medicinal substances. This empirical strategy had already appeared sporadically in medical treatises completed before Shen Kuo's day, but it was not until the eleventh century that it figured prominently in medical literature.

How and why did the empirical strategy of documenting medical practices through personal experience rise to prominence in the Song period? That question is the focus of this book. Although I use the terms "empirical" and "experience" in a philosophical sense, the Western notion of experience had no counterpart in premodern Chinese narratives; for example, Chinese authors did not posit the existence of concepts and knowledge acquired independently from sensory perception. Nor did Chinese thinkers who narrated their personal experience as a strategy for substantiating knowledge mean to claim that sensory perception was the ultimate source of knowledge.[3] The term "personal experience" is used here as shorthand for hands-on practices and sensory perception.

The term "empirical strategy" differentiates documentation through authors' experience as a method of making knowledge *claims* from the use of authors' experience as a source of knowledge itself. Hands-on experience has remained an essential source of medical knowledge. No one would doubt that an author's healing practice and sensory perception in some way inform the knowledge recorded in his medical treatise. Of interest here are changes in the ways of narrating experiential knowledge in medical literature over time and how those changes suited the social and intellectual environment of the day.

The empirical strategy was one of many literary devices that authors deployed to enhance the credibility and reliability of their writings. These devices functioned as persuasion strategies. My concept of "persuasion strategies" is inspired by that of "literary technology," which was developed by the historians of science Steven Shapin and Simon Schaffer in their groundbreaking study of the competing ways through which scientific knowledge claims were legitimized in seventeenth-century Europe. They proposed the concept of literary technology in reference to literary practices through which phenomena produced by experiments with a new instrument of the time, the air pump, were made known to those who were not direct witnesses to its effects.[4] Although the medical authors discussed throughout this book performed no technological experiments, the literary practices they conducted, such as the empirical strategy, function similarly as a means of convincing readers of the factuality of their medical accounts. Through the lens of those authors' persuasion strategies, this book charts changes in competing ways of warranting medical knowledge claims in middle-period China, particularly between the ninth and twelfth centuries.[5]

PERSUASION STRATEGIES AND
THE CHINESE MEDICAL HISTORY

In the history of Chinese medicine, the Song era has been marked by its government's unprecedented involvement in medical affairs. It was in the Song dynasty that distributing medical texts to local officialdom and laymen became a significant means of "educating and transforming" (*jiaohua*) the public.[6] The Song imperial government's sponsorship of medical publishing began in the mid-tenth century, reaching its peak in the eleventh century, when it began printing an array of texts that had been completed before and during the Song era.

The dominant form of printing in imperial China was woodblock printing. This requires less expensive equipment and less capital, thus incorporating images more easily and cheaply than moveable-type printing, which was the preferred form of printing in early modern Europe, where its burdensome capital requirements entailed the centralization of printing centers.[7]

Woodblock printing technology in China had developed in the eighth century but was applied mainly to Buddhist texts. It was after the mid-tenth century, when the Song state was established, that the technology was first used for a wide range of written genres, including medical literature.[8] This wider use made eleventh-century China the world's first print culture.[9] Coexisting with the spread of printing technology, earlier media used for publishing medical literature—hand-transcribed manuscripts (some posted in publicly accessible spaces) and stone inscriptions—continued to flourish, including via the imperial court. In addition to the court, various entities in the Song, including local government officials, degree holders of civil service examinations, physicians, and commercial publishers, printed medical texts. Several regions across China, including Henan, Zhejiang, Jiangxi, Sichuan, and Fujian, produced printed medical books in this era.[10]

While it coexisted with a still-vibrant manuscript culture, as mentioned above, the nascent print culture in the Song era reshaped cultural elites' reading and writing practices, as well as their perception of mass communication.[11] To capture this coexistence, in this book I use the terms "print" and "imprints" only when primary sources clearly indicate that a given text under discussion was printed. Otherwise, I use the term "publish" to refer to any means of distributing texts to the public. Later, in the sixteenth century, printed books, with their significantly lower prices, became the dominant media for transmitting the written word.[12]

The Song imperial court's sponsorship of medical publications was unprecedented. On the one hand, in imperial China there were no institutional qualifications or controls regulating the writing and publishing of medical texts. Ostensibly, any literate and resourceful individual, even if he was not trained in medicine, could collect, compile, and circulate medical treatises to the public. On the other hand, oral transmission within families from one generation to the next or through master-disciple apprenticeships remained significant paths for transmitting medical knowledge. Such esoteric paths of transmission largely reflected the concept that the efficacy of medicine should be transmitted through ceremonies in which masters selected capable individuals and passed down healing knowledge and techniques to them.[13]

Beyond these narrow, circumscribed paths of transmission, there existed other publicly oriented pathways for transmitting medical knowledge. Archaeological excavations in recent decades show that in the Han dynasty (202 BCE–220 CE) some medical texts, in particular formulas, had already circulated among aristocrats and officials with no family backgrounds in medicine.[14] The conspicuous expansion of imperial medical education in the Sui dynasty (581–619) marked the institutional recognition of and engagement with publicly available paths for transmitting medical knowledge.[15] Such pathways decoupled the perceived efficacy of remedies and healing techniques from the specialized paths of transmission that seemed to confine medical knowledge to privileged lineages. The public means of transmission utilized in the Tang dynasty (618–907) extended along paths over which imperial officials posted or inscribed medical texts in publicly accessible spaces.[16] In addition to officials, a growing number of scholarly elites and even some physicians during the transition from the Tang to the Song promoted the dissemination of medical texts as an important public benefit and accordingly published medical texts they collected, edited, or composed.

In the eleventh century, the Song court began printing doctrinal medical texts that had been completed during the Han dynasty. Its efforts stimulated the integration of theories derived from those Han doctrinal texts and healing practice in the Song era. This integration characterizes the Song era as one of three critical transitional periods in the history of medicine in China. These transitions comprise the crystallization of medical theories during the Han dynasty, the integration of doctrinal learning and healing practice under Song rule, and the impact of Western biomedicine since the nineteenth century—a formulation that has been adopted in English-language scholarship on Chinese medicine.[17] Indebted to historians' insights into innovations in Song medical policies, the present study explores how state policies changed persuasion strategies that medical authors deployed, a topic that has received little scholarly attention to date.

Persuasion strategies are useful for examining important turning points in the history of medicine in China. In addition to the empirical strategy, other types were used in medical literature in imperial China. A long-lasting one was citing authoritative sources, especially medical classics that were attributed to semidivine sages.[18] This strategy appeared in the first century CE and continued to be used in later medical treatises, until the authority of classical Chinese medicine experienced a serious crisis in the early twentieth century. Another commonly used persuasion strategy involved asserting the "efficacy" (*yan*) of recorded therapies without specifying who had witnessed the successful outcomes. This appeared frequently in medical treatises composed between the fourth and tenth centuries. After the eleventh century, however, some Song authors, when applying the empirical strategy in their medical treatises, criticized earlier medical authors who did not use it as reckless and earlier medical treatises that did not deploy it as unreliable. Such criticism shows how the criteria by which some texts were judged to be more reliable than others changed over time.[19] The rise of the empirical strategy thereby provides a window through which to view transformations in the construction of textual authority in middle-period China.

The development of and changes in persuasion strategies were intertwined with political-social transitions and epistemic cultures that evolved over centuries and across dynasties. Examining changes in persuasion strategies thus yields a new angle, from which to not only disclose long-term evolutions in Chinese medicine but also unveil relationships between those changes and contemporary epistemic cultures.

Although modern scholarship rarely investigates changes in persuasion strategies *per se*, their findings regarding the development of "medical case statements" (*yi'an*) in imperial China reveal empirical strategies of the time.[20] The study of medical case narratives has not only opened an indispensable window through which to view key social and cultural transitions in China, but it has also become a fruitful site for generating comparative histories of medicine.[21]

Historians often trace medical case narratives back to a biography of an eminent physician, Chunyu Yi (fl. ca. 180–54 BCE). The biography was written by a later historian, Sima Qian (ca. 145?–86 BCE) and published in *Records of the [Great] Historian* (Shiji, ca. 90 BCE). According to this biography, an imperial decree commanded Chunyu to describe his successful prognoses and healing treatments. Chunyu respectfully replied that he always created "examination records" (*zhenji*) after each encounter with a patient.[22] These records did not survive, but presumably they informed the twenty-five medical cases related in his biography.[23] It is perhaps unsurprising that, like Chunyu Yi, many healing practitioners in ancient and imperial China, such as physicians and pharmacists, recorded their healing events for their own purposes and kept their records privately or, at most, circulated them on a limited basis within their families or medical lineages.

During the Song dynasty, a rapidly growing number of authors began to publish medical treatises that related narratives based on their personal experience. What separates those case narratives (such as Shen Kuo's *Good Formulas*) from privately kept medical case records (such as Chunyu Yi's) is that, for an author, publishing a medical text meant attending to a series of issues that are absent from private records. Those include presenting authors' self-images effectively, devising persuasion strategies for selling knowledge claims, and convincing readers of the efficacy of healing practices and medicines. In other words, it was the intention to publish medical treaties that made claims to validity and authority important.

The sixteenth century witnessed the emergence of medical case statements as a new genre on their own. Two early examples are *Sayings of a Female Doctor* (Nüyi zayan, first printed in 1511), and *Stone Mountain Medical Cases* (Shishan yi'an, 1519). In the new genre, medical cases took up most of a text and often attributed cases to only a single healing practitioner. This new genre grew rapidly during the Ming (1368–1644) and Qing (1636–1911) dynasties, which together constitute the late imperial period. Working in this new genre in the late imperial era were physicians who documented and published compilations of their medical cases as supporting evidence of their virtuosity and of the efficacy of a given prescription style or medical "lineage of learning" to which they attached themselves. The production and proliferation of medical case compilations emerged in the context of the competitive healing market and the commercially prosperous book market in late imperial China.[24] In the first half of the twentieth century—the early republican period—when competition between Chinese medicine and Western medicine intensified, Chinese physicians who pursued the standardization and professionalization of Chinese medicine began reconstructing and adapting the genre of medical case collections to the Western medical model of recording individual "disease cases" (*bingan*).[25]

Recent scholarship has noted that the development of the new "medical case statements" genre had interesting counterparts in Europe.[26] Sixteenth-century Europe likewise witnessed the emergence of a distinct medical genre in which case collections became the main content of a text. That genre is known as *observationes*.[27] Scholarship compares the *yi'an* genre with *observationes* in terms of, for instance, the format of the two genres, their association with pharmacological manuals, and "genre awareness" (authors' clear awareness of the case narrative as a new form of medical writing).[28] In contrast to the attention scholars have paid to this comparison, relatively few studies have compared medical case narratives in China with those in Europe before the sixteenth century. This book's contextualized case study of the Song era will facilitate comparative studies of the case narratives in premodern Europe and China.

Deeply indebted to the rich accumulation of scholarship on histories of medical cases in imperial China, this book nevertheless diverges from existing research methodologies by encompassing both physicians' and nonphysicians' medical writings. When tracing medical cases in pre-sixteenth-century China, existing scholarship has predominantly observed physicians' cases.[29] With its focus on how physicians developed a tradition of thinking with cases, such scholarship finds only a handful of medical treatises in which Song physicians wrote and published their medical cases. By taking nonphysicians' medical writings into account, we can see that Song civil officials, both in-service and retired, left ample records of medical cases in their medical treatises.

This book furthermore shifts attention from the late imperial period to the middle period. Previous studies have explored medical case collections as a new genre that began in the sixteenth century, tracing the origins of medical cases in earlier Chinese dynasties. For this retrospective research approach, medical cases discussed before the sixteenth century served as adjuncts to other forms of writing, and no existing compilation consisted of a single healing practitioner's medical cases.[30] But the Song dynasty was not merely an immature stage in the development of the new genre, lacking single-practitioner medical case compilations. Rather, this "lack" was a distinguishing feature of epistemic cultures during that period. Narrations of medical cases by multiple authors reveal important differences between features of epistemic cultures during the Song dynasty and those in the late imperial era with regard to the concepts and applications of empirical evidence.

EPISTEMIC CULTURES IN THE SONG ERA
AND THE HISTORY OF KNOWLEDGE

The history of knowledge, as an extremely broad field, addresses the formulation, circulation, consumption, and application of knowledge, synthesizing multiple strands of scholarship, such as book history, publishing history, intellectual history, and sociology of knowledge.[31] Of importance here are three significant and related changes in epistemic cultures under the Song that bore similarities to the rise of empirical strategies in medical texts during this period, which was both a product of and catalyst for those changes. Scholars have examined these developments predominantly by focusing on notebooks (*biji*, literally, "brush jottings"), travel literature, and "inventories of things" (*pulu*).[32] The authors of such texts comprised primarily degree holders and bureaucrats, whose social groups overlapped with those of many Song medical authors who applied an empirical strategy.

The first change in the epistemic cultures of Song China was the increasing acceptance of knowledge obtained through hands-on experience as worthy of being learned and written down by the literati (primarily bureaucrats, examination degree holders, and scholar-gentlemen). Literati, or scholar-officials, generally referred to as *ru, shi,* and *shidafu*, had constituted the sociocultural elite since the Spring and Autumn Period (770–476 BCE), and maintained their dominant status in imperial Chinese society until the founding of the Republic in 1911. Over the course of these more than two thousand years, the defining composition of the literati changed several times. During the Tang dynasty, they were primarily hereditary clans that dominated political participation and social prestige. The aristocratic clans were weakened by and eventually disappeared over the turbulent course of events that began with the outbreak of Huang Chao's Rebellion (874–84) and continued through the collapse of the Tang empire in 907 and the political fragmentation of the Five Dynasties in the north and the Ten Kingdoms in the south, eventually culminating in the reunification of China with the founding of the Song state in 960.

During the Song dynasty, the expansion of the civil service examination created a new political and cultural elite representing a wider range of social classes.[33] Holding an examination degree or office, rather than representing a hereditary pedigree, became the core mark of the literati.[34] Over the three-hundred-year span of the Song dynasty, the civil service examinations grew increasingly competitive, resulting in an ever-growing number of well-educated men who attempted but failed to pass them. Paralleling the soaring number of educated men without degrees, the central composition of the literati gradually expanded from degree- and office-holding figures to those who pursued scholarship and other socially beneficial achievements. The Song literati meanwhile pursued social eminence through various means, including examinations, landholding, commercial activities, and marriage.[35]

For the Song literati, Confucian classics, histories, and literary works remained essential subjects of "learning" (*xue*). Nonetheless, the soaring number of notebooks, travel literature, and inventories of things that circulated during this period reflected a change in what counted as knowledge in various fields, based on observing and investigating "objects/affairs" (*wu*), which came to occupy a prominent place in the literati's intellectual world. These three types of texts—notebooks, travel literature, and inventories of things—together covered the breadth of extant subject matter. Travel literature in the Song encompassed sightseeing accounts, river diaries, and embassy accounts. Inventories of things presented authors' connoisseurship of groups of specific objects, such as aromatics, flowers, crabs, coins, stones, and alcoholic drinks.

Among the three types of texts, *biji* (notebooks) is the most difficult to define. Modern scholars identify notebooks primarily according to their contents and the ways in which they present data. By this definition, notebooks cover a wide range of choices in subject matter, including medicine, geography, history, reading reflections, anecdotes of famous historical and contemporary figures, uncanny fantastic phenomena, ghost stories, and so forth. Notebooks present "entries" (or items, *tiao*) related to their subject matter in an item-to-item format without any obvious structure organizing them. These two features of notebooks—the wide breadth of topics and the nonstructural mixture of items—are reflected in words constituting the titles of many notebooks, such as "miscellany" (*za*) and "casualness" (*sui* and *man*).[36] Despite these two features, modern scholars acknowledge difficulties in defining notebooks as a genre, because the item-by-item format can also be found in other types of works, such as inventories of things. Bibliographers since the Song dynasty have never reached consensus over the bibliographical category within which to fit "notebooks." Song texts that modern scholars consider notebooks were classified into several bibliographical categories in imperial China, such as historiographies and "tales" (*xiaoshuo*).[37] Reflecting the difficulty involved in defining the notebook genre, the number of extant notebooks produced during the Song era varies in modern scholars' accounts, from 155 based on a narrow definition to 1,103 based on a broader one.[38]

The second change in Song epistemic culture was the growing presence and autonomy of individual authors. Many notebook authors articulated their critical reading and personal verification of the textual and oral information they received.[39] A few literati in the twelfth and thirteenth centuries even claimed that Song authors' verification in notebooks separated Song learning from that in previous ages.[40] Song notebook authors verified received information in various ways, which included critically evaluating it, drawing on textual evidence, accounting for their witnessing of a phenomenon in question, inquiring into interlocutors whose sources of information the authors deemed trustworthy, and documenting informants' backgrounds (such as who witnessed reported events, where, and when).[41]

A term that Song notebook authors frequently used to refer to these various methods of verifying information is "seeing and hearing" (*jianwen*, or conversely, "hearing and seeing" [*wenjian*]). The term "seeing and hearing" additionally appeared in travel literature and inventories of things. In these two types of works, "seeing and hearing" less frequently served as the evidential basis of authors' statements that challenged or rectified information they had received. This term appears widely in the titles, paratexts, and contents of Song notebooks, in which "seeing and hearing" was a broad term and could designate one or multiple methods of acquiring knowledge. Depending on the narrative context, the methods involved could include either seeing and hearing in a narrow sense or broader hands-on experience or document reading, or even all of the above. When used as an indication of knowledge acquisition in Song notebooks, the epistemological focus of the term "seeing and hearing" lies in accentuating "the presence of an individual seeker with epistemic autonomy."[42]

The third change in epistemic culture during the Song involved the increasing intellectual value of the reliability of a given text. The various methods by which Song notebook authors verified received information often promoted the reliability of their notebooks. A growing body of scholarship has characterized reliability as a crucial concern of Song notebook authors. In this scholarship the term "reliability" refers to methods through which notebook authors acquired knowledge that they considered grounded. It also indicated their assurances of the trustworthiness of the information sources on which their notebooks were based, as well as their emphasis on the historical factuality of events they reported.[43]

The foregoing three changes in Song epistemic cultures can all be found in medical treatises that were completed in the Song era. The authors of many Song medical treatises accounted for the knowledge they acquired primarily through hands-on experience, stressing their critical reading and personal verification of the texts they had read and seeking to prove the reliability of their treatises. A close intertextual dialogue existed between medical writings and notebooks during this period. Medical authors and notebook authors often cited and commented on each other's opinions regarding healing affairs. This intertextual dialogue renders the investigation into the foregoing three changes in medical literature indispensable to our understanding of transitions in epistemic cultures in Song China.

Examination of medical literature adds new dimensions to our understanding of the abovementioned changes in Song epistemic cultures and enriches common chronologies of those changes. Historians have concentrated on the development of the three changes in Song China between the tenth and thirteenth centuries. This book is going to trace these changes back as early as the late ninth century—the late Tang period—revealing the continuity in epistemic cultures between the late Tang and the Song, one that has hitherto been explored only minimally.

The prominence of the empirical strategy in medical texts provides particularly effective sources, enabling us to observe the dynamics and tensions between new and conventionally accepted persuasion strategies. Such dynamics and tensions are difficult to analyze in reference to notebooks, because notebooks represent fields of knowledge so divergent that they belonged to no specific genre or knowledge domain and adopted no conventionally agreed-on strategies. In contrast, medical literature developed over a long span of time, beginning at least in the third century BCE, and in the Song era, medical authors deployed the recognized authority of texts and already established persuasion strategies. Song medical literature offers historians rich accounts with which to probe how a new persuasion strategy was introduced into a specific genre, gaining prominence over conventional strategies in that genre. Examining the empirical strategy in Song medical literature thus enables readers to achieve a broader and richer understanding of changes in epistemic cultures in that period.

SOURCES, METHODOLOGY, AND STRUCTURE

This study works mainly with Song notebooks and medical literature. The medical literature I examine consists of texts that would be classified in the bibliographic category that is closest to our present-day understanding of "medicine." The criteria by which texts are counted as "medical literature" has developed and changed over time. In early China, in the bibliographic treatise included in *History of the [Former] Han* (Han shu, completed in the first century), the category is called "remedies and techniques" (*fangji*). This category collects four groups of books: "medical canons" (*yijing*), "canonical remedies" (*jingfang*), "bedchamber instructions" (*fangzhong*), and "methods of becoming immortals" (*shenxian*).[44] From the first century to the Song era, the title of the general category shifted from "remedies and techniques" to phrases explicitly bearing the term "medicine" (*yi*), and includes words such as "healing methods" (*yifang*) and "medical books" (*yishu*).[45] Over this *longue durée*, bibliographers gradually removed many texts previously classified under "bedchamber instructions" and "methods of becoming immortals" from the bibliographic category of medicine. In the Song, two main subcategories constituted the medicine rubric (*yifang* or *yishu*): formularies (*fangshu*, literally, "books of methods," collections of remedies) and the literature of materia medica (*bencao*, literally, "rooted in herbs," collections of introductions to medicinal substances and instructions for their preparation and use). These two subcategories form the primary sources for this book.

Printing technology began to be used to publish writing in medical genres in the Song era, so surviving medical texts from that period outnumber those from earlier ones in Chinese history by a wide margin. The significant number of Song texts that have survived renders that dynasty the first that enabled scholars to chart changes in persuasion strategies in medical literature in meaningful ways. In addition to referencing the medical literature, in order to indicate similar developments in authors' epistemic autonomy and the value of reliability between medical texts and notebooks, I draw extensively on notebooks produced by Tang and Song figures.

When authors of Song medical texts narrated from personal experience as an empirical strategy, they did not rank their own experience above that of their acquaintances—the evidential value of secondhand experience was treated as equivalent to firsthand. When introducing either their experience, their acquaintances', or both, those authors for the most part used the same phrases:

"seeing and hearing" (*jianwen*), "explanatory historical context" (*benshi*), and "facts" (*shishi*). The blurred boundary between experience and the absence of a clear evidential hierarchy indicates a remarkable difference between the empirical strategy and our present-day clear-cut division between firsthand and secondhand experience. The epistemological focus of these terms is not to distinguish firsthand from secondhand experience but to emphasize authors' epistemic autonomy in light of the sheer volume of medical texts circulated during the Song dynasty.

Although Song medical authors did not coin a particular term to refer specifically to their firsthand experience, their empirical strategy can nevertheless be examined historically. Study of Shen Kuo's notebook has shown that we can observe the Song notebook authors' empirical approaches via a close reading of the rich descriptions of their epistemic praxis that they left in their oeuvres.[46] Along the same vein, the Song medical authors' stress on the empirical strategy can be inferred from their explanations for using the strategy and also by the rich narratives they built based on personal experience.[47]

This book consists of four main chapters that focus on four political-social-intellectual contexts in which authors of Song medical texts came to consciously deploy the empirical strategy. Although these chapters cover a period that runs from the fifth into the thirteenth centuries, they focus primarily on changes that occurred between the late ninth and twelfth centuries (the late Tang and Song dynasties). The chapters are sequenced chronologically according to the completion dates of the principal medical treatises scrutinized in each chapter. This arrangement will help us see the chronological development of the empirical strategy in middle-period China.

On the pages that follow, we will see that the prominence of the empirical strategy intersected intimately and consequentially not only with an increasingly distinctive stress on the reliability of a work and on the author's verification and epistemic autonomy but also with a new learning environment that grew out of the medical publishing boom of the Song era. This integration of three fields—the histories of medicine, knowledge, and publishing—through the thread of persuasion strategies compels us to appreciate the production and publication of medical literature as an integral part of the Song literati's epistemic culture. More broadly, this investigation introduces important new perspectives on differences between middle and late imperial epistemic cultures.

INTRODUCTION   *13*

ONE New Criteria for "Good" Medical Formulas

Treating small children whose navels have not been dry for some time, have become red, have developed swelling, and have oozed pus and watery liquid:

Chinese angelica [*danggui*]: Dry it over a slow fire. Grind it into a fine powder.

Put this on the right-hand side on the sick child's navel. Use it frequently, and the child will consequently recover from this disorder. A small child in my household often suffered from a wet navel. Once, this continued for over fifty days. Other remedies were pasted on his navel, but he did not recover. *The Imperial Grace Formulary* collects tens of formulas. We tried those formulas initially, testing each one in turn. But with this formula, one application of the paste made the child's navel dry.

—Shen Kuo, *Su Shen neihan liangfang*, 73.816

THE ABOVE DESCRIPTION of a treatment for a childhood malady represents the general structure of a formula recorded in formularies in imperial China. A formula usually begins with the name of a given remedy or with the names of disorders that need treatment, a description of symptoms, and identification of other disorders to which it could be applied. Such an entry then lists ingredients, methods of processing those ingredients (often in smaller characters), and instructions for administering the remedy. Beyond this general structure are terms attesting to a remedy's therapeutic effects, if a formula author preferred adding them. The precise formulation of the terms would change over time. Before the ninth century most formulary writers briefly noted a medication's efficacy, such as it "having effects"; after the ninth century, such terms came to involve largely narrative accounts of successful outcomes that a given remedy had achieved. These generally included, for instance, a patient's personal background, his or her relationship with the formula's author, and his or her medical history. The new narrative form of describing a remedy's effects soon prevailed in the Song medical literature, illustrated well by the above-quoted example, which comes from the scholar-official Shen Kuo's *Good Formulas* (*Liangfang*) (fig. 1).

In *Good Formulas*, Shen not only frequently promotes a remedy's effects through this new narrative form but also considers this way of disseminating medical information a key element of a high-quality, trustworthy medical formula. He even criticized earlier medical treatises that did not apply this narrative form as unreliable. Interestingly, Shen never received authoritative medical training and thus had no expertise in medicine. In *Good Formulas,* he was never ashamed to admit uncertainty regarding which remedies work more effectively. Such uncertainty is obvious in the abovementioned pediatric formula and in the case narrative by Shen we encountered at the beginning of this book. Growing up in a literati family, he entered officialdom as a clerk at twenty-four years of age. Seven years later, in 1063, he finally earned an "advanced scholar" (*jinshi*) degree—acquired by passing the civil service examination—and then began his colorful bureaucratic career as a civil official. After being sent to the front against the Tanguts and losing a battle on the northwestern border in 1082, all his political ranking was revoked in 1085. He later resided in Run Prefecture (close to present-day Zhejiang and Jiangsu), spending his final years there completing *Good Formulas*.

How far did the elements of qualifying formulas that Shen proposed differ from those mentioned in earlier formularies? What intellectual and social factors built Shen Kuo's confidence—insofar as he was apparently lacking in medical expertise—in proposing such elements and even using them as criteria for the credibility of earlier formularies?

CLAIMING EFFECTS WITHOUT WITNESSING

Throughout the history of imperial China, claiming that recorded remedies had the desired effects had been a significant strategy for building the credibility of a medical treatise. In ancient China, when medical treatises were often attributed to legendary and divine figures, such claims were made by associating the transmission of remedies with those prominent figures. Start-

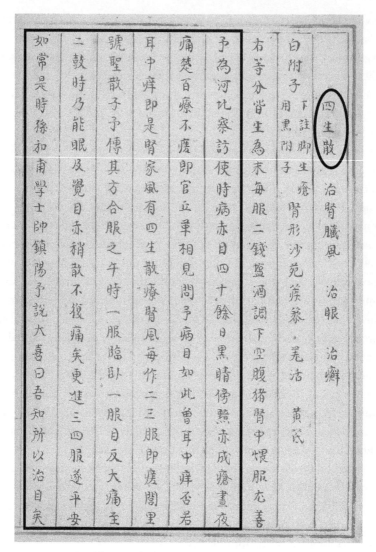

FIG. 1. A medical formula from *Good Formulas*. The first line (vertical) from the right-hand side records the name of the drug remedy (the circled section) and lists the disorders it could treat. The second line from the right-hand side lists the drug's ingredients. The third line from the right-hand side provides instructions for processing and combining those ingredients and applying the remedy. The boxed section presents a healing case that Shen Kuo recalled, detailing when and how he obtained this remedy and used it to treat eye disorders. This formula is preserved in *Good Formulas of the Academicians, Mr. Su and Mr. Shen* (Su Shen Neihan liangfang, a Ming-dynasty manuscript [1368–1644]). Courtesy of the National Central Library, Taipei, Taiwan.

ing in the second century, medical authorship shifted away from this kind of attribution. Medical writers began to identify their names as authors of treatises and sometimes even composed prefaces to express their intentions.[1] Claiming effects for remedies collected in a treatise thenceforth became a way to generate and bolster specific authors' reputations. The primary method of making such a claim shifted from creating a connection with a legendary figure to including the character *yan* in a formula's record. *Yan*, depending on the context, could mean "verify" as a verb, "effective" or "efficacious" as an adjective, or "effect" or "verification" as a noun. It would appear in the names of formulas, such as "a formula for treating foot weakness with magnificent effects," or at the end of a formula record, in phrases such as "having effects," "frequently being effective," "using it [i.e., the given formula] and achieving remarkable effects," "having good effects," and so forth.

The inclusion of *yan* in a medical formula seems to have been less a formulaic expression than an empirical proof.[2] The majority of medical authors between the second and ninth centuries, however, did not specify *who* witnessed the effects. Only a handful described witnesses who had attested to the effects of some of the formulas. These references included their names and personal backgrounds, as well as the dates when the formulas were applied.[3] According to modern scholarship, the first formulary that incorporated authors' medical cases in China is *Essential Formulas Worth a Thousand in Gold, for Emergency Preparedness* (Beiji qianjin yaofang, hereafter *Essential Formulas*), which was completed by the eminent physician Sun Simiao (ca. 581–682), sometime before 659. Sun included twenty-five of his medical cases, involving a variety of remedies, in *Essential Formulas*. Using these to support the efficacy of the formulas he recorded, Sun exhibited an innovative empirical strategy that was rooted firmly in personal experience.[4]

Other examples of formulas incorporating witnesses' information appear in *Mr. Cui's Collections of Essential Formulas* (Cuishi zuanyaogfang), a treatise presumably compiled by a high-ranking civil official named Cui Zhiti (?–681).[5] *Mr. Cui*, for example, recorded how Cui designed a drug remedy to treat diarrhea and cured a dozen people.[6] It also detailed an experience in which a monk assisted with the delivery of an infant, a record that was transcribed from another earlier but now lost treatise, *The Regulating-Qi Formulary* (Tiaoqi fang). The treatise is attributed to a renowned monk, Tanluan, who was active during the Northern Wei dynasty (386–534). In the record, Tanluan used the first-person pronoun to document vividly how he helped Mr. Yang's daughter-in-law deliver a child without incident.[7]

Granted, no reader would doubt that some portion of the effects claimed in formularies for certain medicines derived from the authors' own witnessing or hands-on experience. Authors before the ninth century generally did not, however, identify individuals who testified to the effects of a formula. Sun Simiao's *Essential Formulas* is an example of this practice. Of some 4,000 remedies collected in this formulary, Sun only incorporated twenty-five medical cases. That ratio (0.6%) is surprisingly low, especially when we consider that Sun, as an active and eminent physician of his time, presumably attended a considerable number of healing events. The twenty-five cases must constitute only a small fraction of such events in which he was involved. Sun did not explain the rationale behind his selection of these few cases. The low ratio and the absence of an explanation together imply that in Sun's view, the documentation of those who witnessed the effects of a formula was not instrumental to building a remedy for its reliability.[8]

The scarcity of surviving formularies that were completed before the Song dynasty might be the chief cause of the paucity of records that describe individuals' witnessing the effects of certain formulas. Except for Sun Simiao's two, we have only fragments of the contents of the majority of pre-Song formularies, which are preserved in two large-scale encyclopedic formularies. One is *The Formulary of Secrets and Essentials from the Imperial Library* (Waitai miyao fang, hereafter *The Imperial Library Formulary*), which Wang Tao (702–772) compiled and presented to the Tang court in 752.[9] Another is *The Formulary at the Heart of Medicine* (Ishimpō), which the court physician, Tamba Yasuyori (912–995), compiled between 982 and 984 in Japan and presented to the court in 986.[10] The fragments of information left by those incomplete pre-Song formularies prevents scholars from properly analyzing the portions that explain medical formulas for which there were witnesses who testified to their effects.

In addition to the names of medical formulas, the character *yan* (verify, being effective/efficacious, effect or verification) also appears in formulary titles, where it generally immediately precedes another character, *fang* (methods, formulas, or formularies), as in "collections of effective formulas." Literary scholars and historians have long analyzed book titles when exploring paratexts in European books. Literary scholarship observes that they serve two descriptive functions. One is "thematic," whereby a title signifies the contents, themes, and topics of a given book. Another is "rhematic," indicating its narrative form or genre.[11] Recent scholarship has applied this observation in examining titles of medical publications in imperial China, showing that when the word *fang* appeared in formulary titles, it was used either thematically or rhematically. When it was used thematically, the word should be translated as "formulas" (designating the main content of a book); when it was used rhematically, it should be translated as "formularies" (designating a textual genre that contains formulas and other remedies).[12]

Formulary titles containing the phrase "effective formulas" (*yanfang*) began proliferating in the Era of Division (220–589) and continued to be popular during the Song dynasty. The use of the phrase "effective formulas" in book titles denotes the thematic, not rhematic, qualities of a formulary, because the phrase implies that the remedies collected in a medical treatise were tested and proven effective. Given the fragmentary nature of extant pre-Song formularies, however, it is difficult to examine the degree to which their authors narrated scenarios in which allegedly "effective formulas" achieved their therapeutic objectives. A formulary that gives us a sense of such fragments is *The Formulary that Treats Cold Damage Disorders and Is Bodily Verified* (Liao shanghan shen yan fang). The title suggests that this formulary consisted mainly of formulas whose effects had been attested to, based on the author's personal experience with them. Unfortunately, the treatise is now entirely lost and known only by its title, as listed in the imperial bibliography of *Sui Dynasty History* (Sui shu, compiled by Tang court scholars from 621 to 636).[13]

It is not until the ninth century that we find a formulary that highlighted witnesses to the effects of a formula. The text is titled *Passing on Trustworthy Formulas* (Chuanxin fang, 818) and was written by a civil official, Liu Yuxi (772–842). In his preface to this formulary, Liu indicated that he had verified the effects of all the formulas he collected. He recalled that, in 805, when he was exiled to Lian Prefecture (in Guangdong), the governor of Jianghua County (in Hunan) and his friend, Xue Jinghui, gave him *A Collection of Effective Formulas from Past to Present* (Gujin jiyanfang), which Xue had compiled, and hoped Liu would "complement what this formulary lacks." In response, Liu thereby selected approximately fifty formulas from his box that he had tested. Liu claimed that "all of them have grounds and this is why I used *Passing on Trustworthy* as the title."[14] Although Liu did not specify whether the character *zi* (grounds) referred to the textual origins of those formulas or to sources of information about their effects, the narrative purpose of his compilation favors the latter interpretation. Along this line, the word *xin* (trustworthy) in the formulary title refers to the quality of the sources of information about the formulas' effects.

Moving to the Song dynasty, we find a similar emphasis on the reliability of information sources regarding formulas in *Mr. Wang's Formulary for Broad Relief* (Wangshi boji fang). Its author, Wang Gun, a low-ranking official who was responsible for selling alcohol in Qiantang (in Zhejiang), finished this treatise in 1047. Wang said that he had devoted himself to collecting formulas for two decades, in the process acquiring seven thousand of them. "Those formulas," he declared, "are all transmitted from family documents and obtained from relatives and old friends. They are not received through eavesdropping or oral transmission."[15] Of the seven thousand formulas, Wang selected those that were particularly "essential" (*jingyao*) and known to be effective, compiling them into *Broad Relief*.

The empirical strategy emerged in the seventh century, marking a new persuasion strategy in the formulary genre that foregrounded knowledge rooted in authors' personal experience. With few exceptions, however, the authors of formularies that were completed between the seventh and ninth centuries apparently applied the empirical strategy only rarely. They did not regard the inclusion of information identifying *who* verified a given formula's effects as central to legitimating the reliability of their work. Most of these authors believed that simply declaring that their medical formulas had been used and had proven effective sufficed to establish their reliability. There was no need to document their efficacy by referring to actual cases or patients. I use the term "effective-formula strategy" here in reference to this single means of reliance on formulas known to be effective, thereby distinguishing this strategy from the empirical strategy that Shen Kuo followed in his *Good Formulas*.

NEW CRITERIA FOR THE GOODNESS OF FORMULAS

Questioning the evidential value of the effective-formula strategy, Shen Kuo in his preface to *Good Formulas* proposed various elements of a qualifying and trustworthy formula. One such element is documenting witnesses: "What I call 'good formulas' have to be those of which I have witnessed their effects and then written them down. Hearsay has no role in my identification."[16]

Scholars have regarded this sentence as a path-breaking event in formulary writing and often cite it when examining Shen's empiricism and, by extension, exploring that of Song scholar-officials more generally.[17] But what did Shen mean by the seemingly straightforward term "witness" (*mudu*)? And to what extent did Shen's standard for goodness in formulas depart from that of earlier authors? Because the title of Shen's formulary is *Good Formulas*, when he explains in his preface what "good formulas" (*liangfang*) are, it is difficult to judge at first glance whether he is merely introducing characteristics of formulas that he collected in his formulary or proposing criteria for judging formulas as good in general. Analysis of the structure and content of Shen's preface to *Good Formulas* and a comparison of it with earlier formularies shows that Shen treated the elements of "good formulas" that he mentioned in the preface as criteria for formulas in general.

Shen Kuo's preface to *Good Formulas* is relatively long in comparison with others that were written before or during the Song dynasty. It opens with a lengthy description of what Shen termed "five difficulties" (*wunan*) one might encounter in treating disorders. After describing these, he criticizes earlier formularies for neglecting such difficulties and declares that he collected only formulas the effects of which he had "witnessed." He concludes the preface by explaining his method for listing formulas in *Good Formulas*.

The five difficulties Shen mentions in his preface are "discerning disorders" (*bianji*), "treating disorders" (*zhiji*), "consuming drugs" (*yinyao*), "prescribing medical formulas" (*chufang*), and "differentiating drugs" (*bieyao* or *bianyao*).[18] *Ji*, and other Chinese terms (such as *bing* and *hou*) that indicated what disorders should be treated with medicine, referred to mental and physical issues that are much broader in scope than the term "disease"—in the biomedical category—implies. Medical authors in imperial China seldom used those terms to distinguish clear-cut biomedical categories of ailments, symptoms, syndromes, and diseases. To indicate the wide scope of reference of these Chinese terms, they are more properly translated as "disorders" than as "diseases."

Shen Kuo's explanation for choosing these activities as the five difficulties is so detailed that it occupies almost ninety percent of the preface. The first difficulty involves discerning disorders by examining not only a sick person's pulse pattern but also his or her complexion and "twelve bodily channels." The second difficulty involves treating disorders in accordance with a sick individual's particularities, which might range from age to body size to social status to place of residence and other characteristics, as well as the seasons and the weather when a sick person experienced a disorder, and the progress of that disorder. The third difficulty, "consuming drugs," pertains to tailoring preparation methods to specific drugs; for instance, some were suitable for cooking for a long time or over a strong fire while others were not. The fourth difficulty involves prescribing medical formulas by attending not only to the specific qualities of each ingredient—to avoid cases in which the effects of a drug might be diminished when combined with other medicinals—but also to a sick patient's particularities. The final difficulty, "differentiating drugs," involved discerning between high- and low-quality ones, which was sometimes a function of the geographical features of the places where the drugs originated, the seasons when they were collected, or the methods used to collect and store them.

Concluding his articulation of the difficulties, Shen commented that "the five are merely a sketch. Their intricacy reaches the point that speech cannot express it; their details reach the point that writing cannot record them. How could vulgar persons easily speak of medicine?"[19] Notably, throughout the preface, Shen uses no specific terms to designate the intricate phenomenon toward which the five difficulties gesture—he uses the pronoun "it" (*qi*) only. His silence further manifests his stress on the ineffable nature of the profound healing arts.[20]

Concepts resembling Shen's belief that the subtlety of healing arts defied articulation could be found in the words of the administrator and historian, Sima Guang (1019–1086). He disagreed with the policy of selecting medical officials only via oral tests of their acquaintance with medical classics; he argued that, through the accumulation of experience in treating disorders, "a good physician" (*liangyi*) could examine his success and failure, investigate the essence of healing arts, obtain the arts via his heart, and learn nothing at all via reading ancient texts.[21]

After narrating the profoundness of the healing arts, Shen Kuo juxtaposed his criticism of earlier formularies with elements of good formulas that he proposed: "Those who compose formulas in the world, when mentioning the therapeutic effects of the formulas, often prefer to overstate it. As for formularies like *Thousand in Gold* and *Kept in One's Sleeve*, they are especially full of exaggeration, which makes people dare not to believe those formularies again."[22]

Immediately after these remarks, Shen wrote the sentence quoted at the beginning of this section, announcing that what he calls good formulas were those the effects of which he had "witnessed." After this sentence, he shifts back to his criticism of earlier formularies and then introduces another element of his good formulas:

However, people's disorders are like what I call five difficulties; how could a formula invariably be good? As soon its effects are seen, calling it good; does this method of identifying a good formula bear no difference from marking a boat from which a passenger dropped his sword into a river so as to find the lost sword when he came back to the river again? I thereby detail situations under which a formula had effects at the end of the formula so that one who suffers similar disorders may coincidently match the conditions and implement it.[23]

Taking the preceding two quotations together, we can acknowledge the value Shen attributed to case-based knowledge and his disagreement over viewing effects as a single factor for identifying a good formula. The identification pattern over which Shen disagreed is reminiscent of the effective-formula strategy that prevailed in pre-ninth-century formularies. The two formularies Shen criticized were both widely acclaimed medical treatises of the Song period. *Kept in One's Sleeve* was *The Formulary Kept in One's Sleeve for Every Emergency* (Zhouhou beijifang, or *The Formulary Kept in One's Sleeve to Rescue the Dying*, Zhouhou jiuzu, hereafter *Formulary Kept in One's Sleeve*). Its author, Ge Hong (283–343), was one of the most prestigious scholars and Daoist practitioners of his day. He completed this formulary sometime between 306 and 333.[24] *Thousand in Gold* was a common abbreviation of *Essential Formulas*. As early as 932 but sometime prior to 1064, this formulary had been printed, possibly engraved by a commercial publisher.[25] The Song court edited *Essential Formulas* in 1066 and printed this edited version in the same year.[26]

In addition to mentioning the achievement of therapeutic effects, Shen Kuo proposed two more elements of a good formula. One is an author's "witnessing" its effects, which concerns the standard for selecting formulas to be collected in a given formulary. Another is providing detailed descriptions of situations where a formula succeeded, which concerns the pattern followed for writing the formula. The two elements functioned as proof that the effects of a given formula are not an author's fabrication or overstatement, and as instances of specific circumstances in which a formula would have effects.

From the content and structure of Shen Kuo's preface, we can see that his words regarding the elements of good formulas serve to redefine the criteria for all formulas rather than to introduce features that his book collected. The first indication is the presence of the evaluative rhetoric that he deploys. A comparison of Shen's preface with Liu Yuxi's will help us discern the former's evaluative language. In the latter, the word "trustworthy" that Liu used in his formulary's title established that the sources of information from which he had learned of the effects of his formulas were well grounded. Throughout Liu's preface, he avoids commenting on the trustworthiness of other formularies. Like Liu, Wang Gun, in his preface to *Broad Relief,* merely sounds a note of caution concerning the sources of information that confirm formulas' effects without commenting on other formularies' sources. In contrast, Shen Kuo not only compared his proposed elements of good formulas with those in two other famous formularies, but he also evaluated and criticized the two. In so doing, in my reading, Shen featured his proposed elements not merely as characteristics of his own formulas but also as alternative standards for those that deserve high praise.

The structure of Shen's preface further indicates that he regarded his proposed elements as criteria for good formulas. The preface starts with his articulation of the five difficulties that one might encounter when trying to achieve therapeutic results. Only after spending several paragraphs expounding on these difficulties did Shen then launch into his critique that the authors of earlier formularies employed effects as the single standard of good formulas and propose his own elements. The question "How could a formula inevitably be good?" at the end of the aforementioned quotation nicely encapsulates the gist of Shen's entire preface, that is, the contingent nature of formulas' effects in the realm of medicine.[27]

Shen's lengthy description of the five difficulties, through the structure of the preface, illustrates the contingent nature of the effects of formulas, hence helping his readers understand the defects in the conventional criteria for a good formula and appreciate why his offer superior alternatives. To better illustrate the structure of Shen's preface, we must compare contexts where the contingent nature of formulas' effects is mentioned in the preface and where it appears in *Essential Formulas.*

The principle that effective treatment required taking all the contingent factors associated with disorders into account was an entrenched idea that existed well before Shen's *Good Formulas.* In the early seventh century, for example, Sun Simiao had already remarked in the very first chapter (*juan*) of his *Essential Formulas* on the principle that prescriptions should be adapted to patients' particularities. That chapter comprises nine sections. The names and sequences of the nine sections show that Sun discussed this principle in the context of explaining how to learn and practice medicine; in sequence, they are: "1. Great Physicians' Learning Practices," "2. Great Physicians' Diligence and Honesty," "3. Brief Examples of Treating Disorders," "4. Diagnosing," "5. Prescribing," "6. Applying Drugs," "7. Combining Compounds," "8. Consuming Drugs," and "9. Storing Drugs."[28]

Sun introduces, in the second section, difficulties encountered when attempting to discern disorders and, in the third, proposes a general strategy according to which a prescription should be modified in accordance with the geographic particularities of places where a sick individual had stayed. Sun's introduction to such difficulties and the corresponding strategy, within the framework of the nine sections, serves in part as a guide to practicing medicine. By contrast, although the five difficulties in the preface to *Good Formulas* concern a similar prescription principle, immediately following this exposition, we encounter Shen's proposal that detailing the circumstances in which a formula has succeeded is one of two elements of a good formula. The sequence of Shen's narrative clearly manifests the context in which he talked about the prescription principle as the proper template for documenting a formula rather than as a general rule of healing practices.

Shen Kuo thus proposed three elements of a good formula: indicating a remedy's tested effects, documenting an author's "witnessing" of its effects, and narrating situations where it succeeded. The three are criteria for qualifying formulas. The first was already commonplace in formularies completed before Shen's day; the other two are relatively new. Shen's advocacy of the criteria thereby places more empirical weight on the word *yan* ("effective" or "effects") in formula writing than it had borne before.

LIMITS OF EXPERIENTIAL VOCABULARIES

Good Formulas comes down to us in an altered form. It was added to a collection of Shen's other writings concerning medical affairs and formulas, and to prose writings about medicine that the leading literary figure of Shen's day, Su Shi (1037–1101), composed. The expanded version is known as *Good Formulas of the Academicians Mr. Su and Mr. Shen* (Su Shen neihan liangfang, hereafter *Su's and Shen's Formulas*).[29] The earliest indication of the existence of *Su's and Shen's Formulas* comes from a privately compiled catalog of books, *Memoirs of Reading in the Jun Studio* (Junzhai dushu zhi, ca. 1151–87, printed in 1180–84).[30] Over the course of the twelfth century, *Su's and Shen's Formulas* superseded *Good Formulas*, becoming the predominant version. The declining circulation of Shen's original version, as historians have noted, is evident in changes in introductions to this formulary in the other two privately composed catalogs in the Song era. One is *The Suichu Hall Catalog* (Suichu tang shumu), which was completed by You Mao (1127–1194). Another is *Zhizhai's Annotated Catalog* (Zhizhai shulu jieti), which was written by Chen Zhensun (1179–1262). Both catalogs introduce *Su's and Shen's Formulas* without mentioning *Good Formulas*.[31]

The received version of *Su's and Shen's Formulas* consists of 252 items, 172 of which historians have identified as left by Shen Kuo.[32] Among those, 143 are accounts of therapies. Historians generally agree that the 143 items were drawn from Shen's original *Good Formulas*. The contents of some of the 143, however, differ markedly from Shen's criteria for writing a good formula. In the preface, Shen stresses having a "witness" to the effects of a formula as a criterion for selecting it for *Good Formulas*. In the main text, nonetheless, relatives or acquaintances of Shen attested to the effects of many formulas.[33]

Sources that attest to the effects of formulas in the main text, some of which Shen himself notes explicitly and some of which I infer, can be classified into eight types and sequenced on the basis of how closely each resembles Shen's firsthand experience. Of the 143 items, 30 do not offer information sources for the effects of the remedies in question. Many offer multiple types of information sources.

The first type of source is Shen himself, after applying a remedy to himself or to others and achieving therapeutic effects.[34] The second type is when Shen documents how he "personally saw" (in Shen's words, *qinjian* or *mujian*) the effects of a remedy.[35] These first two types correspond to our modern notion of having a witness, but in total these types account for only 24 of 143 items. The third type of source is when Shen gave a remedy to someone and that person found it effective (13 items).[36] Shen's own relatives represent a fourth type, constituting the second largest portion of the 143 items (28).[37] The fifth type derives from people whom Shen documents in *Good Formulas* as friends or at least people to whom he had spoken personally (11 items).[38] The sixth type is listing the names of persons who had been treated effectively but with whom Shen does not indicate having any particular relationship, which forms the largest portion of the cases (52 items).[39] In the majority of the cases that I classify as of the third, fourth, fifth, and sixth types, it is difficult to know for certain whether Shen learned of the effects of their treatments by witnessing them himself or by hearing from those individuals after the fact. The seventh type of source involves secondhand knowledge, that is, hearing from third parties that particular formulas had treated patients effectively (1 item).[40]

26   CHAPTER ONE

Finally, in some cases Shen learned of the effects of a formula by reading about them (7 items).[41]

Let us consider several explanations for the inconsistency shown in the abovementioned statistics. One is that *Su's and Shen's Formulas* encompassed records that Shen had not collected in *Good Formulas*. If we were to count only formulas belonging to the first and second types as those drawn from *Good Formulas*, the number would be twenty-four. This number, however, is remarkably lower than the current scholarly consensus suggests, according to which most of Shen's formulas in *Su's and Shen's Formulas* came from *Good Formulas*. This apparent conflict with the current scholarly consensus reduces the likelihood that this explanation is true.

Another factor that might explain the inconsistencies among the sources of information that Shen claimed in the preface and what is reflected in the main text is that, because in the former he already mentions witnessing the effects of formulas that he had collected in *Good Formulas*, he did not believe it was necessary in the main text of the formulary to account for scenarios in which he had witnessed a given therapy succeed. If that had been the case, the various types of sources that Shen noted in individual formulas would turn out to have been nothing but his arbitrary choices.

A more grounded explanation of the inconsistency is that Shen saw no fundamental differences in evidential power between validating a formula through personal experience and doing so by reference to others whose information sources he deemed reliable. This explanation can be supported by the typical narrative focus in Shen's formulas: the historical factuality of the case histories. One example comes from a formula for the Costus Root Pill (Muxiang Wan). In the formula, Shen offers two case histories in which the pill succeeded.[42] The first involved narrating a healing event in which his elder brother, Shen Pi, was the patient. The second depicted a case that involved Shen Kuo himself.

Shen Pi led soldiers in pursuit of bandits in Zhangpu (around present-day Zhangzhou city in Fujian), and all of the soldiers were suffering from "intermittent fever" (*nüe*); the Costus Root Pill cured them. Shen Pi was presumably in Zhangpu in 1077, when he was director-in-chief of the Fujian circuit.[43] In the same year, Shen Kuo was first provisional commissioner of the State Finance Commission and was then assigned to Xun Prefecture (in Anhui).[44] He by no means was able to witness the effects of the pill in Fujian. Shen Kuo said nothing about why he narrated his brother's healing event before narrating his own. This silence denotes that the narrative focuses not on differences between firsthand and secondhand experiences but rather on the historical fact that the pill achieved its effects in specific circumstances.

A relatively indirect piece of evidence indicating that Shen Kuo was willing to accept secondhand testimony as readily as his own experience of the effects of the formulas he included in *Good Formulas* is that the equivalence between seeing and hearing was widespread across genres in Song China. This equivalence is exemplified in pharmacological texts and notebooks. As I observe in the next chapter in light of more specific evidence, the authors of notebooks and pharmacological writings in the Song era would use what they saw or heard from others whom they deemed reliable to expand on or challenge existing pharmacological reports. One example of this practice can be found in Shen's notebook *Brush Talks from Dream Brook* (Mengxi bitan, hereafter *Brush Talks*).[45] When accounting for what they saw and heard, those authors rarely prioritized the former over the latter. A shorthand phrase that those authors frequently employed to refer to such information sources is "seeing and hearing" (*jianwen*, or conversely, "hearing and seeing" [*wenjian*]). Granted, the phrase "seeing and hearing" expresses equal appreciation of those two knowledge sources far more explicitly than the phrase "witness" (*mudu*), which Shen employs in his preface.[46] Despite the difference between the phrases, however, it is difficult to ignore the fact that Shen demonstrates the same equation between seeing and hearing in his contributions to *Su's and Shen's Formulas*.

The main texts of Shen's formulas that *Su's and Shen's Formulas* collected show that his "witnesses" actually encompass experiences of both the author and others. When presenting formulas, Shen draws no clear line between the evidential power of his experience and that of others. Moreover, in Shen's description of his or others' experience, the narratives do not focus on differences between firsthand and secondhand experience. Instead, he emphasizes historical factuality, specifying circumstances in which a given remedy had proven effective. This equation of the evidential power of authors' seeing and hearing also appeared frequently in notebooks and pharmacological writings during the Song dynasty.

SHEN KUO'S EPISTEMOLOGICAL PROPENSITY

From its preface to its presentation of arrays of formulas, *Good Formulas* exhibits the same epistemological predilections as Shen Kuo's other famous work, *Brush Talks*, which he finished sometime between 1088 and 1095, a period overlapping his composition of *Good Formulas*. *Brush Talks* contains records of a wide range of subject matter, including administrative issues, music, calligraphy, painting, natural phenomena, medicine, and so forth. Many of the records fall into domains of knowledge that we now classify under the rubric of science, such as chemistry and astronomy.[47] The records concerning his discoveries of scientific knowledge place Shen ahead of his time and render him a well-known polymath in modern China.[48]

Although he was a keen explorer of multiple domains of knowledge, Shen strongly doubted the human capacity for fathoming and articulating the ultimate principle of the universe. In *Brush Talks*, the doubt can be seen most clearly in an entry in which he argues that, in terms of calendric calculations, a human designer cannot precisely predict the "degree" (*du*) of movement of celestial bodies. Shen adds that "people in the world who speak about such a number capture only its coarse vestiges. However, there is an especially intricate number that cannot be known via calendars."[49]

Notably, as in the case in which Shen used only "it" (*qi*) in reference to the inarticulable profoundness of the healing arts underlying the five difficulties, in this quotation Shen again fails to employ specific terms to denote the intricate number. His opinion here of the limited predictive capacity of human-designed numbers to calculate calendrical dates resembles his belief in the limited capacity of vocabularies to transmit medical knowledge. Considering that humans were unable to expound on the profoundness of the universe, Shen passionately observed and recorded particular "things" (*wu*, including objects and affairs) that he believed derived from the profoundness of the universe. In *Good Formulas*, Shen elaborated on the contingent nature of a remedy's effects and detailed the conditions in which a formula succeeded, but made no attempt to address prescription strategies related to the profoundness of the healing arts. In *Brush Talks*, for example, he recalled how he anticipated the pattern of "circulated qi" (*yunqi*) by observing changes in the natural environment, such as the strength of the wind, whether it was rainy or sunny, and whether the grass and trees were flourishing or withering.[50] Shen's interest in observing and recording particular things is also evident in various projects that he worked on during his bureaucratic career in the 1070s, such as supervising hydraulics, reforming calendars on the basis of his astronomical knowledge, and surveying the Song state's border with its northern Khitan neighbor, the Liao state (907–1125).[51]

When composing *Good Formulas* and *Brush Talks*, Shen tended to present his records of particular things in a nonsystematic manner. In *Brush Talks*, he arranged the records, which covered a broad range of subject matter, in an item-to-item layout without an obviously systematic scheme for organizing them. This manner of presenting knowledge in *Brush Talks* is understandable insofar as most notebooks adopted a similar approach. The two features together made notebooks an ideal written platform for authors interested in recording various findings that were not systematic or rich enough to constitute an independent book. In comparison, the nonsystematic presentation of knowledge in *Good Formulas* is especially noteworthy. Among the historical sources I have found, Shen is the first author who explicitly admitted to listing formulas in his formulary in no particular sequence. He says in the preface to *Good Formulas* that he arranged "sections out of sequence; as long as I was able to obtain a formula, I recorded it and gave it to others."[52]

In formularies completed before and during Shen's time, the conventional organization of formulas involved grouping them by the types of disorders that a given one could treat. The search logic behind this organizational approach was that a reader would first find a section corresponding to specific disorders or symptoms from which people were suffering and then search for an applicable formula in that section.[53] By diverging from such an organizational scheme, the nonsequential listing that Shen deliberately employs in *Good Formulas* was far more challenging for a reader who was eager to find a formula quickly. Shen scribed this unusual arrangement to his eagerness to share effective formulas with the sick, which he claimed left him no time to classify them systematically. Here, Shen's explanation turns the nonsequential presentation of formulas into a manifestation of his benevolence.

Shen's epistemological propensity determined the contents and presentation formats of both *Brush Talks* and *Good Formulas*. His epistemological approach included the denial of the human capacity to fathom and articulate the profoundness of the universe, an intense interest in observing and recording particular things, and a preference for presenting knowledge in a nonsystematic manner. This trifold propensity, especially in regard to the first two, helps to explain Shen's emphasis on the contingent nature of the therapeutic effects of formulas and on documenting situations in which a formula proved effective. In addition to his epistemological propensity, other external social and intellectual contexts of Shen's day likewise fostered the emergence of his new criteria for good formulas.

30 CHAPTER ONE

SONG MEDICAL GOVERNANCE

Before losing the northern half of its territory to the Jurchen Jin state (1115–1234) in 1127 and rebuilding its regime in the south, the Song state, which is known as the Northern Song (960–1127), engaged itself with medicine, education, and public welfare more actively than any imperial government before or after did.[54] The Northern Song government extended the Medical Academy (Yixue) from its capital to the prefectural level and produced a massive number of medical treatises. It frequently disseminated those treatises and drugs to laypersons across its territory as a form of state relief during epidemics and as an innovative means of educating common people. It also launched many campaigns against the perceived unorthodoxy of healing customs in the south, such as a preference for shamans over medicine. During this period, providing drugs and medical texts to common people was beginning to become a central means of demonstrating Song rulers' benevolence, exhibiting the state's authority, and legitimizing its rule.[55] Provision of medical care became more politically meaningful than ever before.

Modern historians have studied this conspicuous expansion of state involvement in medicine in the Song era, which they characterize as medical governance or medical activism.[56] Some policies associated with medical governance were integral to a series of reforms designed to resolve social and bureaucratic problems that the Northern Song court undertook, which include the short-lived Qingli Reforms (1043–45) and the influential New Policies (1069–85). From the execution of the New Policies through the fall of the Northern Song in 1127, proponents and opponents of the policies conflicted with each other, spawning venomously factionalized politics. Medical activism nonetheless outlived those factional conflicts. Historians have observed multiple motives that encouraged the long-lived regime of medical governance in the Song era. One was the Song emperors' personal interest in medicine, especially in collecting medical formulas.[57] The other motives included the desire to earn high financial profits from selling drugs to imperial subjects, political and medical demands associated with rampant outbreaks and epidemics, and the military's need to maintain the well-being of soldiers stationed on the borderlands. The last motive was an absolute necessity, considering that the Song state existed under constant military threat from its powerful neighbors.

Few policies that historians regard as integral to Song medical governance exerted influence as lasting as the government's medical publishing projects. Their profound influence derived mainly from their qualitative and quantitative outcomes. Over the course of 350 years before the Song era, the imperial court commissioned only five medical treatises, whereas, in its 160-year reign, the Northern Song court cut woodblock versions of at least twenty-five medical texts.[58] The court's editions of those texts often became the oldest that we have now, and many of the twenty-five texts are still used in today's traditional Chinese medicine (TCM) curricula in China.

The Song government's devotion to distributing medical writings marks the first time in Chinese history that rulers attempted to "educate and transform" (*ji-aohua*) the common people by disseminating medical knowledge, especially in textual form.[59] This devotion arose at the very beginning of the Northern Song dynasty, when the court was still waging bloody campaigns to reunite China. In 973, the founder of the dynasty, Emperor Taizu (r. 960–976), initiated a textual project that involved editing pharmacological texts and compiling them into the encyclopedic *Newly Established Materia Medica in the Kaibao Regime* (Kaibao xinxiangding bencao). In 974, Taizu asked the same editing team to revise this text, in a year that overlapped with his 974–76 campaign against the Southern Tang state (937–976), whose capital was located in present-day Nanjing (in Jiangsu). The court claimed that it converted the two pharmacological texts into woodblock-printed editions soon after their completion.

In 978, approximately two years after the conquest of the Southern Tang, Taizu's younger brother and the succeeding emperor, Taizong (r. 976–997), began a textual project that involved compiling an encyclopedic formulary. This formulary, finished in 992, bore the title *Imperial Grace Formulary of the Great Peace and Prosperous State Era* (Taiping shenghui fang, hereafter *Imperial Grace Formulary*) and collected as many as ten thousand medical formulas. In 981, Taizong issued an order to compile another encyclopedic formulary.[60] Completed in 986 or 987 and titled *The Formulary for Magnificent Healing and Universal Relief* (Shenyi pujiu fang), that work survived at least until the end of the Northern Song dynasty but is now lost. It was impressive in terms of sheer volume, comprising as many as a thousand chapters.[61]

Roughly overlapping with the compiling and printing of these two formularies were numerous battles fought against the Liao, the biggest northern threat to the Song at that time. The court carved the two grand formularies into woodblocks immediately after their compilation. *The Imperial Grace Formulary* became one of the most often-cited in the Song era.[62] After 1005, when the

Song campaigns reached a peaceful conclusion with the Chanyuan Covenant with the Liao, thereby securing its rule over China, the court's projects that involved compiling and editing medical literature reached a peak during the mid-eleventh century.[63]

In addition to the court, local government officials were also enthusiastically producing and publishing medical literature. Their discourses on the advantages of distributing medical texts resembles those the court issued. Both often appealed to the political implications of distributing medical texts as a tool for educating the general population as well as to the ethical value of such distribution as a manifestation of benevolence.[64] The media that the court and other officials used to publish medical texts ranged from scribbled forms to stone inscriptions to woodblock printing.

Changes in the use of printing technology in the late eleventh century further increased the accessibility of imperially commissioned medical texts and expanded their readership. In the eleventh century, court-sponsored medical publications were accessible predominantly to imperial physicians, students receiving imperial medical education, and scholar-officials whose positions placed them in the capital. The Directorate of Education (Guozi Jian, literally, the Directorate of Sons of the State) was the chief institution in charge of printing court-compiled texts. Before 1088, the directorate's medical imprints were printed in large characters. These required a greater investment in paper and ink, resulting in prices that put them out of reach for lay physicians. In 1088, noticing the restricted availability of these imprints "in the public" (*minjian*), the Song court began to print medical literature in small characters to reduce prices. These helped increase the availability of Song court–compiled medical literature.[65] From the second half of the eleventh century onward, imperially printed books spread steadily in greater quantities and at lower prices.[66]

THE RISE OF LAY MEDICAL READERS

The Song court's and other officials' devotion to distributing medical treatises facilitated and extended the public transmission of medical knowledge. This eventually enabled the number of self-taught medical learners to reach a critical mass for the first time.[67] Public availability favored self-taught learners, who collected medical texts and then edited and compiled them into "new" medical treatises. Indeed, these became an important group of medical writers in the Song era. The presence of autodidacts as medical authors indicates that no sharp boundary between "professional" writers and "amateur" readers existed in that period. Readership for medical literature was extended to include people whom authors had not known or contacted in person. Knowledge was transmitted to such readers primarily in written formats rather than, as had traditionally occurred, through physicians' families and in master-disciple lineages, where oral instruction and practical demonstration played vital roles. In comparison, then, with traditional disciples and those who learned medical care from older members of their families—all of whom could learn through written texts as well as personal contact with experts—the expanding group of self-taught learners depended largely on written words.

Of these, many were lay medical readers, literate people who had learned about medicine primarily by reading texts without the assistance of mentors and often found it difficult to design treatments without consulting those texts. Such readers already existed before the Song dynasty, but they gained greater visibility in Song writings. For instance, in the preface to *Good Formulas*, Shen Kuo says that he hoped his detailed descriptions of circumstances in which formulas succeeded could enable one who was suffering from a similar disorder to map the condition and apply the formula with good results. Shen's words sketched out a type of medical reader who was able to read medical literature but unable to design treatments without consulting it.

The same type of reader appears in almost the same context in Wang Gun's preface to *Broad Relief*. Before each section of his work, Wang detailed symptoms, a patient's "pulse pattern and breath" (*maixi*), or the origin of a particular disorder. In so doing, Wang envisioned "one who did not understand medicine, who can meticulously read the detailed accounts and then adapt it to making therapies." To be sure, it is plausible to assume that a formulary author might exaggerate the population of lay readers to enhance the authoritativeness of his knowledge or to justify the publication of his new book. This possibility nevertheless does not preclude the existence of such readers.

In addition to mentioning lay readers frequently in prefaces, medical formulas, and postscripts to medical treatises, authors in the Northern Song era began depicting in more specific and vivid terms the circumstances in which such readers consulted medical texts. One case in point comes from the pediatric formula we encountered at the beginning of this chapter. In the formula, Shen Kuo notes how he or his family members tried to find a remedy that would be effective for the sick child by administering formulas collected in *The Imperial Grace Formulary* one by one. Such a trial-and-error approach was a staple of lay medical readers. The act of consulting *The Imperial Grace Formulary* moreover reveals their use of treatises commissioned by the Song court.

Other examples concerning the expanding presence of lay medical readers appear in diagnostic instructions that Shen offered in *Good Formulas*. Those rarely required special skills and could be comprehended and carried out easily. For instance, when recommending the use of a Minor Construct-the-Middle Decoction (Xiao Jianzhong Tang) to treat "depletion cold" (*xuhan*) and pain in one's abdomen, Shen instructed his readers to identify the depletion cold simply by pressing a patient's abdomen: if the patient felt pain immediately but less when stronger pressure was applied, this sensory perception would support a diagnosis of depletion cold in the abdomen.

Following the foregoing instructions, Shen quoted sentences that he attributed to Zhang Ji's *Treatise on Cold Damage Disorders* (Shanghan lun, ca. 202–17, hereafter *Treatise on Cold Damage*) to specify another method for identifying conditions under which the Minor Construct-the-Middle Decoction could be applied. That required that readers be familiar with pulse diagnosis, an advanced diagnostic skill that differed entirely from Shen's easy-to-apply method. The quotation reads: "When the yang pulse pattern is 'rough' (*se*) and the yin pulse pattern is 'string-like' (*xian*), the method of treating acute pain in one's abdomen is to first administer this decoction."

Here we see technical terms associated with pulse diagnosis, which was an important technique in classical medicine in imperial China and should be distinguished from pulse-taking in present-day Western biomedicine. The latter focuses on the rapidity and regularity of a patient's pulse, whereas pulse diagnosis in classical Chinese medicine applied to a variety of conditions that involved relatively subjective tactile perceptions on the part of practitioners. When conducting pulse diagnosis, practitioners typically placed their fingers (usually three) on the underside of the patient's forearm below the wrist. Imperial Chinese medical texts described the tactile perceptions gained from pulse diagnosis using a rich array of verbs and adjectives, such as "sinking" (*chen*), "floating" (*fu*), and "deficient" (*xu*).[68] It would take years, even decades, for a diligent medical trainee to master the art of pulse diagnosis. In comparison, the procedure and results of the first diagnostic method that Shen noted were so straightforward that any literate layperson could follow them.

The increasing presence of lay medical readers in Song writings indicates to a certain degree the growth of this readership in the Northern Song era. Extant data do not allow us to gauge the specific extent to which the lay medical readership had grown. Nevertheless, reported figures indicating how many candidates were taking civil service examinations provide some sense of the growing number. Examination candidates constituted an important group of people who were literate enough to read medical literature or might be interested in medicine. The frequent regional trips that those candidates took between their hometowns and examination venues created a need to learn about medicine or at least to be able to apply basic self-treatments on the road. Of course, not every examination candidate had such an interest or was able to access medical literature. We do however see that, starting in the eleventh century, some candidates abandoned their fruitless attempts to pass the examinations and chose to earn their living practicing medicine.[69] It is probably safe to suppose that many of the candidates consulted medical texts.

One physician who had been an examination candidate, Dong Ji (fl. 1102–1117), even wrote the first formulary devoted to travelers in China, *The Formulary for* [*Ones Staying at*] *Travel Houses, a Provision of What Is Essential* (Lüshe beiyao fang). Travelers whom Dong mentioned as the targeted readership of his work included officials who traveled from a current administrative position to the next one, usually every three years, and "guests" (*ke*) on the road, whom Dong did not specify but might have included merchants and examination candidates.[70] Dong's formulary did not survive, but Qing officials reconstructed one chapter (*juan*) from the Ming court–compiled encyclopedic work, *Great Compendium of the Yongle Era* (Yongle dadian, 1403–8). Differing from Shen Kuo's *Good Formulas*, the lone extant chapter of Dong's formulary collected no narratives of healing events. But some of his formulas did concern disorders that might have occurred during trips, such as encountering coldness or heat stroke.[71] Dong's frequent trips as an examination candidate might have inspired him to compose this formulary.

Civil examinations during the Song dynasty, to be very brief, took place every three years on three levels: the prefectural, the departmental (at the capital, for those seeking advanced-scholar degrees), and the palace (for degree holders to be assigned to their bureaucratic posts according to their ranks). In the early eleventh century, there were approximately 20,000 to 30,000 candidates standing for prefectural examinations, but the figure soared to 79,000 a century later and exploded to 400,000 by the middle of the thirteenth century.[72] When gathering at prefectures for forthcoming examinations, candidates often were more easily able to access medical texts than they would have been in their

36   CHAPTER ONE

hometowns. Even if only half of the candidates in any given round of tests could access and read medical texts, the number is still considerable.

In imperial China, a lay medical reader, if he continued to improve his healing skills, could later proclaim himself a physician and practice medicine as the source of his livelihood. During that era, no institutional qualifications or training served as the gatekeeper to determine who could practice as a physician, nor did any controls differentiate qualified practitioners from incompetent ones. Anyone capable of practicing certain healing skills could call themselves "physicians" and set their own fees.[73] Becoming a physician became easier with the increasing availability of medical publications from the Song period onward. This ready availability helped increase the number of self-taught medical practitioners in the Song era.[74] Dong Ji, for example, was an examination candidate and self-taught medical learner before staking his livelihood on medicine and composing *The Formulary for Travel Houses*. Bearing this in mind, here the phrase "lay medical readers" serves as shorthand to refer to medical learners with limited healing skills, reflecting the possibility that skill levels changed over time.

When Wang Gun and Shen Kuo touted the benefits of their detailed descriptions of situations in which a given formula succeeded, they both mentioned the benefit of helping their readers judge the suitability of the remedies they were recommending. On the one hand, helping such lay readers, who were unable to design suitable treatments without consulting formularies, might contribute to the authors' justification for writing a new formulary. On the other hand, the extended public transmission of medical literature and a critical and ever-growing mass of examination candidates in the Song era provide a solid foundation for the existence and expansion of an audience of lay medical readers. Starting in the eleventh century, descriptions denoting such readers appeared with greater frequency.[75]

SCHOLAR-OFFICIALS, THE NEW MEDICAL AUTHORITIES

In 1057, the "military affairs commissioner" (*shumi shi*) Han Qi (1008–1075) submitted a memorandum in which he suggested that Emperor Renzong (r. 1022–1063) order "Confucian officials" (*ruchen*) who understood medical texts and imperial physicians to work together to examine and distribute an array of medical texts: *Divine Pivot* (Lingshu), *Grand Basis* (Taisu), *A-B Canon* [*of Acupuncture*] (Jiayi jing), *The Divine Farmer's Classic of Materia Medica* (Shennong bencaojing, hereafter *The Divine Farmer's Classic*), *Essential Formulas*, and *The Imperial Library Formulary*.[76] Historians have dated the establishment of the Bureau for Editing Medical Texts (Jiaozheng Yishuju) to Han Qi's memorandum.[77] Historians have proposed that the bureau was established as rampant epidemics were breaking out, between 1023 and 1063; the parallel timing suggests that the purpose of founding the bureau was to edit medical texts that would be useful in fighting epidemics.[78] From 1057 to 1069, it compiled one pharmacological encyclopedia and edited ten medical texts. No evidence indicates that the bureau submitted texts after 1069, which suggests the end of the project. The bureau-edited medical texts went beyond serving as textbooks for imperial medical education because the court promptly printed at least nine of the eleven for the purpose of distributing them widely to the public.[79] The establishment of the bureau represents the peak of the Song court's investment in distributing medical texts. After it ceased operations, the court never again launched such a large-scale project related to medical publications.

It is noteworthy that the court assigned Confucian officials, rather than medical ones, the task of supervising the editing projects that the bureau conducted, which institutionally recognized scholar-officials' authority over the editing of medical texts. Before such assignments were made, there was a long-standing practice whereby non-medical officials compiled and annotated medical texts in private hands. At the institutional level, however, when the Western Han court was for the first time in Chinese history (between 26 BCE and 7 BCE) compiling a catalog for the imperial library, which was titled *Seven Catalogs* (Qilüe), it assigned a "medical attendant" (*shiyi*), Li Zhuguo (fl. ca. 26 BCE), to edit books concerning "remedies and techniques" (*fangji*), and the infantry commandant Ren Hong to edit military texts.[80] These assignments were clearly based on the editors' expertise in specific domains of knowledge.

In the eleventh century, court officials forcefully asserted that, regardless of the domains of knowledge to which texts that the court was going to edit belonged, only civil officials in "academies and institutes" (*guange*) should be in charge of editing projects.[81] As shown in relevant memoranda left by court officials at the time, their decision reflected the belief that text editing was not only an administrative duty that officials in academies and institutes should carry out but also a process by which the officials cultivated a broad spectrum of learning.[82] The bureau's basic procedure for editing medical texts involved first collecting multiple renditions of a given treatise, then comparing the contents

38 CHAPTER ONE

of those renditions, and finally teasing out the best possible words or phrases where discrepancies occurred; this was the same procedure that officials in academies and institutes conducted when editing Confucian classics.[83]

Scholar-officials' newly recognized medical authority reflected their capacity to decide which medical writings were useful or significant enough to be edited and then distributed by the court. This authority is evident in the administrative power by virtue of which they could suggest to the emperor which earlier medical treatises were worthy of the state-sponsored editing projects. The Bureau for Editing Medical Texts was founded in accordance with an edict by Emperor Renzong; however, Renzong left us no edict in which he specified which texts the bureau should edit. Instead, many were nominated in officials' political documents, as exemplified in the abovementioned memorandum issued by Han Qi. This point is made in a preface as well: when its staff finished editing Zhang Ji's *Treatise on Cold Damage*, the bureau composed a preface to the edited version. At the end of it is a list of those who were responsible for the editing, all of whom were scholar-officials rather than medical officials. The preface notes that "the state decreed Confucian officials to edit and correct medical texts . . . We considered that, regarding the urgency required by hundreds of disorders, none is more urgent than cold damage. Now we first edited Zhang Zhi's *Treatise on Cold Damage*."[84] This sentence indicates that it was Confucian officials in the bureau, rather than medical officials, who bore the responsibility for deciding which medical texts would be edited.

Only after understanding the medical authority granted to Confucian officials through the establishment of the bureau can we understand the weight of the prefaces they wrote for the bureau-edited *Essential Formulas*. This version, which was completed in 1066, includes both a preface and a "post-preface" (*houxu*). The two end by listing the names of Confucian officials in the bureau, the first three of whom are Lin Yi, Gao Baoheng, and Sun Qi. The earlier draft of the two prefaces was written by another Confucian official, Su Song. Historians have compared the two prefaces with those of Su Song thoroughly, and my discussion here focuses on how they praise *Essential Formulas*.

The four prefaces all cited the advantage of the breadth of textual references that Sun Simiao included in his *Essential Formulas*. For instance, Su Song complimented the formulary for its "profoundness and broad coverage."[85] Lin Yi and other officials also applauded it for encompassing references "drawn from as early as the invention of writing to as late as the Sui dynasty. It did not fail to collect either any classics or formulas. It amassed what numerous healing currents secretly valued." Another advantage that Lin Yi's preface noted is that, regarding its formulas, "none of them cannot perfectly verify their effects."[86] Su Song additionally appreciated that fewer than one in ten medical texts that were completed between the Han and Tang periods survive to his day; only *Essential Formulas,* "whose beginning and end roughly appear and is especially a complete book," remained available.[87]

The three advantages of *Essential Formulas* that the four prefaces praised were the broad coverage of its references, the effects of its formulas, and its longevity (having remained intact for a long time). The first two also appear in the bureau's prefaces to other medical texts that it edited. For instance, in the preface to the edited *Treatise on Cold Damage,* officials cite the historian Huangfu Mi (215–282), who praised it because the application of its formulas "frequently had effects."[88] In the preface to the edited *The Imperial Library Formulary,* officials praised Wang Tao for "collecting the important parts of formulas belonging to numerous currents," a judgment that agrees with the first recognized advantage of *Essential Formulas.*[89]

Interestingly, the above officials' praise of *Essential Formulas* contrasts sharply with Shen Kuo's criteria for good formulas.[90] The two had divergent opinions regarding the appropriateness of applying phrases that remark on the universal effects of a formula as praise. Shen clearly opposed this application. Officials in the bureau, while they accepted the contingent nature of a formula's effects, felt more comfortable than Shen with employing such phrases. Shen moreover differed from officials in the bureau in terms of the scope of the references or formulas that a formulary contained. If an author collected formulas whose effects had been proven only by himself or by his acquaintances, the number of formulas and types of disorders that his treatise covered was inevitably limited. The limited number of formulas and the correspondingly limited coverage of disorders is reflected in Shen's *Good Formulas.*

No textual evidence suggests that Shen Kuo had read the four prefaces to *Essential Formulas.* On the basis of Shen's bureaucratic career, however, I suspect that he at least knew that the bureau edited *Essential Formulas;* his criticism of this treatise therefore could be regarded as an implicit challenge to other Confucian officials' standards for selecting medical texts. The period during which Shen was an official in academies and institutes overlapped with part of the period during which the bureau fully functioned. In 1066, when the bureau submitted *Essential Formulas* to the emperor, Shen was the "editorial assistant for books at the Institute for the Glorification of Literature" (*bianjiao Zhaowen*

40 CHAPTER ONE

Guan shuji). He was appointed the "proofreader in academies and institutes" (*guange jiaokan*) in 1068. Within a month of that, though, he left the position following his mother's death. Insofar as the period during which Shen was an official in academies and institutes overlapped with the year when the bureau edited *Essential Formulas* and the court printed it in 1066, it would be surprising to learn that he never knew at that time that the bureau had submitted the formulary to the emperor.[91] Considering that Shen presumably knew that the bureau edited *Essential Formulas*, his choice of that book as an example that merited criticism may not be simply a response to this treatise's popularity at the time; rather, it may be also a product of his implicit disagreement over Confucian officials' standards regarding which formularies should be edited and distributed by the court.[92]

BEFORE THE NINTH CENTURY, the predominant persuasion strategy used in a formulary was to note that the recorded formulas were known to be effective. Formulary authors who applied this strategy rarely viewed noting *who* attested to the effects of a formula as central to its being deemed good. Diverging from those earlier authors, Shen Kuo in *Good Formulas* criticized that strategy and proposed two new criteria: an author's "witness" to the effects of a formula, and case narratives depicting situations in which the formula succeeded. We should not, however, jump to the conclusion that Shen elevated the role of firsthand observation in writing formularies. An analysis of *Good Formulas* shows that the "witnessing" that Shen upholds in his preface actually encompassed information sources drawn from both his and his acquaintances' personal experience. The wide range of information sources that the term "witness" represents indicates that Shen saw no fundamental differences between testimony based on his own experience and that based on the experience of people whose information sources he deemed reliable. Rather than differentiating between firsthand and secondhand testimony, Shen's "witnessing," along with case narratives, focused on proving the historical factuality that a formula had demonstrated effects. It is the historical factuality, rather than authors' expertise in medicine, that underpinned the credibility and reliability of *Good Formulas*.

Scholars have analyzed the distinction between firsthand observation and secondhand experience extensively in analyzing claims to knowledge in the history of science and medicine in premodern Europe. Their findings reveal a perplexing absence of distinct terminology indicating firsthand observation, an absence reminiscent of what we have encountered in the preceding investigation into Shen Kuo's phrase "witness" and into medical texts and notebooks of his day. In ancient Greek, the Hippocratic physicians recognized firsthand observation as a source of information.[93] Nonetheless, within their corpus, there existed no specialized language that denoted observational practice. What modern scholars have translated as "to observe" does not correspond to any single consistently used vocabulary element. Even as late as the fifteenth century, formulary authors still did not seem to embrace the notion that firsthand experience should be demarcated from secondhand evidence and be clearly labeled accordingly.[94]

Shen's proposal for new criteria for *Good Formulas* derived from his epistemological propensity as much as from changes in his surrounding social and intellectual circumstances. He doubted the human capacity to capture the ineffable profoundness of the healing arts. This doubt sparked his keen interest in observing and recording particular things that he thought originated in profoundness, such as specific conditions in which a formula achieved therapeutic effects. Shen attributed his advocacy for describing such conditions to his aim to help readers map them onto a given sick person. This then would enable readers to find a formula that was suitable for that person's particular bodily condition. Shen's targeting such readers as the chief audience of *Good Formulas* paralleled the ever-growing population of lay medical readers in his day.

Imperial recognition of scholar-officials as a group with medical authority helps us understand Shen Kuo's confidence in and engagement with listing criteria for good formulas. This imperial recognition owed largely to the eleventh-century court's project of editing and printing formularies, which established the Bureau for Editing Medical Texts and assigned Confucian officials to lead the projects. This assignment institutionally recognized Confucian officials, and by extension all scholar-officials, as a group in which it invested medical authority. Their recognized areas of authority included correcting medical documents, as well as deciding which medical texts were useful and important enough to be disseminated across China by the government.

Although Shen assertively promoted the new criteria for good formulas, their influence on later Song medical writing is no more obscure than that of *Brush Talks* on later Song notebooks. As scholarship has noted, Shen had already used reliability to assess *Brush Talks*; nevertheless, no authors of later notebooks that were completed in the Southern Song era identified Shen as a significant contributor to this trend when applying reliability as a standard of assessment in their writing. What historians can best say in terms of the influence of *Brush Talks* is that Shen "provides a solid precedent in the immediate past that Southern Song literati were eager to invoke."[95] The same could be said of the role that *Good Formulas* played in the development of medical writing: although many later Song medical authors likewise documented witnesses to a remedy's effects and wrote case narratives to prove them, they rarely attributed this practice to Shen Kuo.

The obscurity of the influence of *Good Formulas* on Song medical writing by no means impugns the historical significance of that treatise. The treatise signals, in the domain of medical genres, the coming of a new configuration of knowledge production featuring unprecedentedly wide dissemination of medical literature through government and private publications, a soaring population of lay medical readers, and scholar-officials as a group invested with medical authority that for the first time received state support and institutional recognition.

The emergence of this configuration owed largely to Song medical governance, yet its impacts were much more profound than the Song emperors and officials intended.[96] One product is *Good Formulas*. This formulary offers us a rich account of how a new pattern, in which authors documented empirical evidence pertaining to a formula's effects, emerged in response to this configuration. Twenty years after the completion of *Good Formulas*, a medical author collected his case narratives in his pharmacological work. Its emergence against the new configuration is the subject of the next chapter.

TWO Textual Claims and Local Investigations

A woman delivered a child in a cold month, and cold qi entered her birth gate. Her abdomen below the navel then became distended with fullness. She and others dared not touch the distension. This was "cold amassment" [*hanshan*]. A physician was about to treat her with a Resistant and Withstanding Decoction [Didang Tang], saying that the woman had "blood stasis" [*yuxue*]. I taught him that it was not a pertinent treatment, and that she could consume Zhang Zhongjing's Lamb Meat Decoction, with reduced water. She consumed two dose of the Lamb Meat Decoction and recovered.

—Kou Zongshi, *Bencao yanyi*, 16.104

THIS MEDICAL CASE appears in an entry on "black ram's horns" (*guyang jiao*) that was included in a pharmacological manual, a genre that rarely preserved case narratives. This manual, *Elucidating the Meaning of Materia Medica* (Bencao yanyi, hereafter *Elucidating the Meaning*), was written by a low-level official, Kou Zongshi, the administrator of the Revenue Section of Li Prefecture (in Hunan). No evidence suggests that Kou had received solid medical training.

In addition to documenting medical cases in this manual, Kou also, remarkably for the time, recorded his observations of medicinal substances he encountered during his extensive travels as a civil servant. He compared his observational findings with entries in earlier pharmacological collections, and he creatively placed his medical cases and observational findings side by side with his introduction to those substances. After completing *Elucidating the Meaning* in 1116, he submitted it to the court the same year. First printed in 1119, *Elucidating the Meaning* later became one of the most widely printed pharmacological collections during the Song dynasty.

Modern scholarship has noted Kou's extraordinary emphasis on his observational findings, attributing this to his individual epistemological propensity and to being influenced by the neo-Confucian concept of "investigating things" (*gewu*).[1] However, two crucial factors in Kou's employment of the empirical strategy in *Elucidating the Meaning* have remained underexplored. First, scholar-officials at the time exhibited heightened interest in documenting their investigations into putatively regional phenomena about which they had read and heard. Their investigations involved a broad range of subject matter, including climatic features, topography, famous natural and historical sites, social customs, indigenous creatures, and local products. The trend toward covering regional phenomena was already burgeoning in the late ninth century and continued into the Song era. Second, the government of Emperor Huizong (1082–1135, r. 1100–1126) designed an array of policies to elevate the status of medicine.

DEPARTING FROM EARLIER PHARMACOLOGICAL TEXTS

What we know about Kou Zongshi today comes primarily from his oeuvre. This includes *Duke Lai's Glorious Loyalty* (Laigong xunlie), a collection of both imperial-issued and privately composed memorialized writings addressed to the grand councilor Kou Zhun (961–1023). Kou Zongshi reportedly proclaimed himself Kou Zhun's great-grandson.[2] Unfortunately, *Duke Lai's Glorious Loyalty* did not survive, and no corroborative evidence can prove that Kou Zongshi was Kou Zhun's descendent. Another, and more solid, source of information about Kou Zongshi's life comes from entries scattered throughout *Elucidating the Meaning*. According to these, Kou had traveled extensively during his official career: besides staying in Li Prefecture (in Hunan), he had been a magistrate of Wushan County (in present-day Long County, Shaanxi), and was once positioned in Kaifeng (in Henan) as well as Luoyang (in Henan) and Shun'an Military Prefecture (in Hebei).[3] Over more than ten years of official travel, he observed medicinal substances and asked locals about them, which informed his work when he collected his investigations into *Elucidating the Meaning*.

The introduction to *Elucidating the Meaning* reveals that Kou composed this treatise in keeping with both a long-term practice, in which private authors wrote pharmacological collections, and a contemporaneous tendency in which Song private authors composed new works in response to state-commissioned pharmacological encyclopedias. The earliest recorded such encyclopedia was *The Divine Farmer's Classic*, which dates to the late first or second century BCE and became the foundation for subsequent pharmacological collections. Its original text no longer exists but is partially preserved through a later annotated edition, *Collected Annotations on the Classic of Materia Medica* (Bencaojing jizhu, hereafter *Collected Annotations*). The author of *Collected Annotations*, Tao Hongjing (452–536), a prestigious figure in Daoist schools and officialdom, grew up in a family that practiced the administration of drugs for at least three generations.[4] He compiled a pharmacological collection when staying at Mao Mountain (in Jiangsu) over two periods—ca. 492–504 and 514–36. *Collected Annotations* was frequently cited as a benchmark for pharmacological knowledge during later dynasties.

Between Tao Hongjing's and Kou Zongshi's times, both individuals and the Tang and Song courts compiled pharmacological collections. Between 657 and 659, the first government-compiled pharmacological encyclopedia in the world, *Newly Revised Materia Medica* (Xinxiu bencao) was produced. By mass-producing it, the Tang court conveyed a clear message that it had brought the natural and medicinal resources across the empire under control. The Song court compiled far more pharmacological encyclopedias than the Tang court did. After *Kaibao Materia Medica* (Kaibao chongding bencao) in the tenth century, the Song court conducted new compilation projects and produced *Supplemented and Annotated Divine Farmer's Materia Medica in the Jiayou Regime* (Jiayou buzhu Shennong bencao, 1057–61, hereafter *Jiayou Materia Medica*) as well as *Illustrated Materia Medica* (Bencao tujing, 1058–62). Magnificent in scale, *Jiayou Materia Medica* introduced 1,082 medical substances and drew references from a wide collection of texts as a central persuasion strategy.[5] Both it and *Illustrated Materia Medica* are now lost, coming to us only through quotations in other Song pharmacological collections.[6]

Based on *Jiayou Materia Medica* and *Illustrated Materia Medica*, Song readers soon began compiling commentaries and new pharmacological collections. For instance, a physician, Chen Cheng (fl. 11th century), combined and annotated them both to create *The Expanded Divine Farmer's Materia Medica and Illustrated Materia Medica* (Chongguang buzhu Shennong bencao bing Tujing, 1092). Kou Zongshi's compilation of *Elucidating the Meaning* is part of the Song authors' response to the state-commissioned pharmacological encyclopedias. It is presented in two parts. The first includes the first three chapters of the treatise and presents Kou's opinions on medical theories and

46 CHAPTER TWO

healing cases. The second, which comprises the remaining seventeen chapters, contains some 473 items that introduce medicinal substances. Supplementing and correcting entries in *Jiayou Materia Medica* and *Illustrated Materia Medica* was the principal objective of Kou's work.

While exemplifying both the abovementioned long-term practice and the contemporaneous tendency, Kou's *Elucidating the Meaning* departs from earlier pharmacological works in four respects: its reliance on empirical strategy, the informal style of its entries, the conspicuousness of its argumentation, and the connection between pharmacological knowledge and "coherence" (*li*) .

The empirical strategy permeates *Elucidating the Meaning*. In Kou's words, he "examined statements of numerous authors and compared them with the facts."[7] Kou does not specify to which "facts" he referred, but if we consider the entries that constitute *Elucidating the Meaning*, we can see that he was referring to his first-person narratives.

Before *Elucidating the Meaning*, even pharmacological treatises containing entries recording authors' firsthand experience occupied only small portions of them. For instance, Tao Hongjing recorded his enquiry from "market people" (*shiren*) regarding drugs in *Collected Annotations*. No extant pharmacological treatises that preceded Tao's work contained such information about authors' firsthand experience. This thus marked the emergence of the empirical strategy in pharmacological texts as a medical subgenre (i.e., annotations). Later, Chen Cangqi (fl. 713–741) in his *Collecting the Omissions of Materia Medica* (Bencao shiyi, ca. 739, hereafter *Collecting the Omissions*) also accounted for his observations and inquiries by citing "dwellers on the mountain" (*shanren*) when describing local medicinal substances.[8] Among the approximately 600 annotations that Tao wrote and the 970 entries in Chen's work, however, only a handful of entries reflected the empirical strategy.[9]

In addition to the prominent visibility of its first-person narrations, *Elucidating the Meaning* is further distinguished from the great body of pharmacological works that had been completed before the twelfth century by the informal style of Kou Zongshi's entries.[10] Under the typical format, an entry provides information about a given medical substance in the following order: its "flavors" (*wei*), its "qualities" (*xing* or *qi*), whether it has "potency" or "toxicity" (*du*), its "main indications" (*zhuzhi*, important therapeutic usage), provenances, and seasons of collection. Other commentaries are then appended to the foregoing descriptions, often chronologically. These came from earlier pharmacological works produced over a period beginning during the Han dynasty and extending to the authors' time. That there were layers of commentaries indicates the crucial role that textual sources played in producing drug-related knowledge. Although not all entries in pharmacological collections follow this format perfectly, they always include at least some of the abovementioned elements.

Consider, for example, Kou Zongshi's entry on black ram's horns, which varied considerably from the typical format. The entry first notes that black rams could be found in Shaanxi and "east of the Yellow River" (*hedong*), describes their external characteristics, and compares them with the horns of other kinds of sheep and rams. The entry then suddenly shifts to note that Zhang Zhongjing treated cold amassment with a decoction of fresh ginger and lamb meat and that anyone who had consumed it had recovered. This note is followed by the medical case translated at the opening of this chapter.[11]

The format of this entry differs from typical formats in both pharmacological collections and formularies. Kou mentioned nothing about the quality or flavor of black ram's horns, which were fundamental elements of pharmacological entries. Neither did he append the medical formula for the fresh ginger and lamb meat decoction, as Shen Kuo did in his formulary, *Good Formulas*. Kou also had no intention of explaining medical vocabulary for his readers. For instance, Zhang Zhongjing is the "style name" (*zi*, or courtesy name) of Zhang Ji (ca. 150?–219?), the author of *Treatise on Cold Damage*.[12] With no drug recipe or explanation, readers would have found it difficult to treat cold amassment by consulting this entry alone. It seems that Kou did not mind this.

Another illuminating entry that illustrates Kou's informal style is an item on fishing cormorants (*luci*):

Fishing Cormorants. Tao Yinju [i.e., Tao Hongjing] said: "This bird does not produce eggs. It spits its brood out of its mouth. Today people call this bird 'old water crow.' It nests on big trees in large crowds. The cormorants have regular places where they rest, and after a long time the trees wither because the droppings of the birds are poisonous. Pregnant women do not dare to eat them because the birds spit their brood out of their mouth." Chen Cangqi additionally said: "To achieve easy delivery, when the time has come, let the delivering woman hold one of the birds." This contradicts Tao. I served as an official in Li Prefecture. Behind my office, a large tree stood. In its top there were some thirty or forty nests of these birds. Day and night, I observed them. Not only were they able to have intercourse, but also their eggshells, which were spread all over the place, were greenish in color. How could they spit their brood out

48 CHAPTER TWO

of their mouths? This has never been questioned or investigated. Apparently, it was the mistake of listening to hearsay.[13]

This quote represents one of the typical narrative patterns in *Elucidating the Meaning*: Kou would first indicate discrepancies or unclear records involving medicinal substances that he found in earlier works (including pharmacological collections, formularies, works of literature, classics, and histories). He would then describe how he verified those records by observing something or asking locals about the substances in question, writing down what he found. Occasionally, he would add his own criticisms of earlier authors who had not examined what they had read or heard. As for this quotation, the text Kou criticized is Tao Hongjing's *Collected Annotations*. In this entry, none of the abovementioned typical elements appears—only Kou's assessment and verification. The absence of such typical components is common throughout *Elucidating the Meaning*. Even when some of Kou's entries include them, they are not presented in the conventional sequence. In contrast, Tao Hongjing's entry on fishing cormorants in *Collected Annotations* follows the typical format: his entry first introduces alternative names and main indications for the excreta, and then the cold quality and main indications of the cormorants' heads, and finally methods of consuming the heads for therapeutic purposes.[14]

The absence of typical components from Kou's work cannot be attributed to his unfamiliarity with them, given that the great number of pharmacological collections cited in *Elucidating the Meaning* attests to his awareness of them. This absence is better understood as a reflection of his preference for informal styles of documenting pharmacological knowledge.

The much wider range of genre-mixing in *Elucidating the Meaning* serves as another indication of its informal style. This is exemplified by its combination of medical cases and entries in pharmacological manuals. Before *Elucidating the Meaning* appeared, few pharmacological collections had incorporated medical cases. In contrast, Kou recorded a considerable number of his medical cases in both the "prefatory examples" (*xuli*) section and the main text of his manual, innovatively integrating the medical case subgenre into the pharmacological one as a persuasive strategy.[15] This feature likewise reflects the atypical format and informal style of *Elucidating the Meaning* as a pharmacological treatise.

Such a departure from the typical format at first glance makes Kou Zongshi's entries seem similar to Tao Hongjing's annotations in *Collected Annotations*. However, a crucial difference between the two is that Kou's entries make up an independent book, whereas Tao's annotations are individually appended to each relevant entry taken from previous pharmacological collections. It is possible that Kou similarly meant to produce an exegetical work: when he submitted his manual to the court in 1116, he might have expected further work to be conducted to separate and align his commentaries in each entry with the corresponding entry in *Jiayou Materia Medica*.[16] Unfortunately, we have no further textual evidence that would inform an assessment of this hypothesis. However, we know with certainty that *Elucidating the Meaning* was first printed as an independent book in 1119 by Kou Zongshi's nephew, Kou Yue, the magistrate of Xie County in Xie Prefecture (in Shanxi).

Argumentation pervades most of *Elucidating the Meaning*. Issues subject to this practice include judging whether an accurate match has been made between an object or affair and its linguistic expression, ensuring that testimony is trustworthy, verifying the existence of a putative phenomenon, and providing the rationale behind the application of a substance. Judging terminological matches, corroborating testimony, and providing rationales were crucial elements of Kou's findings, often determining what he calls the "coherence of a substance" (*jueli*, literally, "its coherence").[17] When Kou could establish the coherence of these three factors related to a given substance, the coherence of the substance was also established.

The entry on "jade spring water" (*yuquan*, reputedly a source of healing) illustrates Kou's argumentation involving a match between an object or affair and its linguistic expression. In the first part of this lengthy entry, he juxtaposes textual collation with his puzzlement regarding earlier pharmacological entries on jade spring water. For instance, Kou notes, *The Divine Farmer's Classic* said that jade spring water originated in a valley in the Lantian region (in Shaanxi) and can be "picked" (*cai*) in any season. Immediately following this citation, Kou is puzzled: no spring exists in the Lantian valley nowadays, and the verb "pick" never referred to collecting spring water either in antiquity or in the present day. *The Divine Farmer's Classic* moreover mentioned consuming a five-*jin* dosage of jade spring water. Kou refuted this statement, claiming that neither ancient nor contemporary medical formulas used the term "*jin*" to characterize dosages of water. He furthermore indicated that numerous authors' explanations of jade spring water focused on the character "jade" and circumvented the word "spring water." Tao Hongjing said that it was called "jade spring water" because this type of jade could "turn into a watery form." If that were the case, Kou wondered, the object should have been named "jade water" (*yushui*)

50 CHAPTER TWO

instead of "jade spring water." He comments that earlier understandings and explanations of jade spring water "after all did not rise to the coherence of a substance." Here it was the seamless match between a substance and its name that warranted the finding of coherence.

Kou's explanation of the meaning of "jade spring water" occupied the middle part of the entry. He opened this part with an assertive answer to the above-mentioned puzzlement, declaring that the word "spring" should be rendered, in conventional vocabulary, a "thick fluid" (*jiang*). Kou then deployed various means of validating his declaration. For instance, he claimed that "five *jin*" did presumably refer to jade in the thick fluid. Picking jade and making it into thick fluid was what was "definitely without doubt." He also argued that this vocabulary mistake stemmed from the fact that the names of a given medicinal substance were omitted or misconstrued during the long-term transmission of pharmacological texts from ancient times to what was then the present day. Kou offered textual evidence of such mistakes as examples. To prove that the term "jade-thick fluid" (*yujiang*) was actually used, Kou cited texts containing this term from *Daoist Canons* (Daozang jing) and sentences containing a similar term, "precious jade-thick fluid" (*qiongjiang*), from a poem written by the talented poet Li Shangyin (813–858).[18]

In the final part of this entry, Kou remarked on his two fruitless "field studies" regarding what jade spring water was. He visited the Jade Spring Temple in Jingmen Military Prefecture (in Hubei). In the temple, there was a spring whose water exhibited "no difference from normal spring water" and had no therapeutic efficacy. He also visited another Jade Spring Temple, which was located on Wan'an Mountain in Xiluo (Louyang City, Henan). He went to that mountain twice, asking monks at the temple about a jade spring. None could answer him. In front of the temple, though, there was a spring, which again exhibited "no difference from well water." In this entry, Kou's central method in supporting his argument was to collate textual sources, reason critically and logically, and present the results of his local investigations.

The entry on fishing cormorants illuminates arguments over the existence of a purported phenomenon as a subject of Kou's discussion. In that entry, his observation served as the single piece of evidence against Tao Hongjing's statement. The entries on fishing cormorants and jade spring water both demonstrate the centrality of the empirical strategy to establishing authorial reliability. This centrality is additionally evident in Kou's criticism of Tao's uncritical acceptance of received information.

Kou's criticism of writers for accepting information uncritically is best seen in two entries. In the entry on stonecrops (*jingtian*, literally, high sky or making heaven luminescent), he indicates that, given that Tao used the phrase "it was said" (*yun*) to describe a stonecrop growing in Guang Prefecture (in Guangdong) that was "three to four times wider than the width of two arms around," it was apparent that Tao did not "personally see" (*qinjian*) the stonecrop, but had merely heard about it. Kou commented that "it was [the product of] Tao's relaxed listening."[19] Another example is the entry on moles (*yanshu*), in which Kou claimed that Tao believed moles lived in mountains and forests, were as big as buffaloes, looked like pigs, and produced their young through the dropping of seminal fluid on the ground. Kou wondered: even if the beasts Tao depicted were indeed moles, no one had ever seen moles producing their young in that manner. Kou concluded, "Tao recklessly trusted [the information] to this degree."[20] The three entries together (on fishing cormorants, stonecrops, and moles) clearly emblematize not only Kou's emphasis on witnessing purported phenomena but also his refutation of the practice of writing down hearsay as a persuasion strategy, one Tao used to his own satisfaction in *Collected Annotations*. This emphasis and refutation in turn justify Kou's enthusiasm for conducting local verification of pharmacological information that he read and heard.

Regarding in-depth explanations of a phenomenon as a topic of Kou's argumentation, one example comes from the entry mentioning "soil made of eastward walls" (*dong bitu*).[21] Kou used this entry to illustrate how he established the coherence that previous authors had failed to establish. It begins with a medical formula that includes this substance and a citation drawn from *Collecting the Omissions*. The citation reads, "Collecting soil made of eastward walls, for the soil was often dry." Kou then launched into a series of self-questions and answers. The first question was: because "soil made of southward walls" (*nan bitu*) was similar to soil made of eastward walls, insofar as both are exposed to sunlight and are often dry, why not take that soil? The answer was: soil made of eastward walls constantly received early sunlight first. Kou said, "Sunlight was the true fire of Great Yang." The subsequent question was: why not take soil made of southward walls at noon, but take soil made of eastward walls in the early morning? The answer was that at the moment the fire ignited (i.e., the sun rose), its qi was strong. This is why soil made of eastward walls taken in the early morning was of higher therapeutic efficacy than soil made of southward walls taken at noon. Kou here additionally drew supporting

52   CHAPTER TWO

evidence from *Basic Questions* (Suwen), a medical canon that was attributed to the ancient legendary sage-king Yellow Emperor, presumably compiled in the Han era, and later heavily edited, printed, and endorsed by the Song court in the eleventh century.

The final question was how one could know that "sunlight was the true fire of Great Yang." Kou replied with an easy experiment: placing wormwood (*ai*) in the center of a beam of sunlight, which was reflected by water or by a bronze mirror with a sunken center, after which the wormwood would catch fire. Throughout this entry, the methods with which Kou validated his answer encompass logical reasoning (on a foundation of cosmological concepts, such as yin and yang), drawing on textual evidence, and verifying information empirically (burning wormwood with sunlight).

In contrast to Kou, whose argumentation pervades *Elucidating the Meaning*, not all of the authors of earlier pharmacological works felt comfortable putting forward their own arguments. Admittedly, some included explicit argumentation, for instance, by giving their opinions about the pronunciation and "flavor" (*wei*) of a given medicinal substance.[22] Other authors of pharmacological works, however, preferred setting references drawn from multiple texts side by side under a given entry. Even when there were discrepancies in the references, the authors rarely judged which one was more accurate. A typical example of this propensity to present eclectic sources without judging their relative value is *Illustrated Materia Medica*, which was compiled by the Song court, which claimed that one of its aims was to provide guidelines for processing and applying medicinal substances. Nonetheless, the compilers of *Illustrated Materia Medica* explicitly stated that, when contemporaneous accounts of a given medical substance differed from records found in earlier pharmacological texts, they would keep both.[23] This policy of not judging which of two differing accounts should be trusted hindered *Illustrated Materia Medica* as an ultimate source for codifying pharmacological knowledge.

Empirically verifying received information, in addition to critically evaluating and reflecting that information, drawing textual evidence, and reasoning logically, constitute the four fundamental methods in Kou Zongshi's practice of argumentation. Through them, Kou justified his findings. In certain entries, he depicted such findings as coherence (*li*), which was a common but polysemous word in Chinese intellectual narratives. In *Elucidating the Meaning*, li refers primarily to a penetrating understanding of a given medical substance. Such a thorough understanding, as shown in the entries on jade spring water and soil made of eastward walls, involved fathoming the rationale behind the naming of a medical substance as well as confirming its therapeutic efficacy and designing the corresponding prescription strategy. Kou claimed that, "without investigating and verifying the coherence of a substance, treating disorders would not only waste efforts but also eventually fail to save lives."[24]

Kou's pursuit of coherence resulted from a very practical concern about therapeutic efficacy, but he had little interest in connecting coherence to moral reflections or in harmonizing it with *li* for other purposes. In this sense, Kou's investigation into medicinal substances and his pursuit of coherence diverged from the neo-Confucianists' intellectual agenda that drove explorations of *li* as a means of cultivating the qualities of a moral human being. Cheng Hao (1032–1085) and his brother Cheng Yi (1033–1107) characterized this agenda as "investigating things and attaining knowledge" (*gewu zhizhi*), conceptualizing *li* as a feature of all objects or affairs, which were connected with each other across the world. Therefore, all *li* is one *li*. A learner could continue investigating *li* in one object or affair and extending it to another. During the process of extending coherence in this way, the learner would eventually attain ultimate and unitary coherence and acquire the qualities of a moral person.[25] Kou never directly linked this agenda with his own pursuit of coherence.[26] The term *jueli* (its coherence) that Kou used was not his invention, as it had appeared frequently across earlier histories and literary works. During Kou's time, the Cheng brothers' teachings circulated primarily among their disciples. The central government even suppressed the brothers' teachings during the Chongning reign (1102–1106). It was not until two hundred years later, when the government endorsed neo-Confucianism, that the synthesis of neo-Confucianism and medical theories emerged in the medical literature.[27]

Four features thus distinguish *Elucidating the Meaning* from earlier pharmacological collections: the high degree of visibility of first-person narratives, the lack of the typical established components of pharmacological collections, the pervasiveness of a deliberate practice of argumentation, and the connection between pharmacological knowledge and *li*. Notably, the first three appear more frequently in notebooks that date to the late ninth century, especially in their authors' entries on local investigations into regional phenomena about which they had read or heard.

LOCAL INVESTIGATIONS IN THE NINTH CENTURY

The innovations that distinguish *Elucidating the Meaning* were part of a far broader and longer-lasting trend in which scholar-officials from the late ninth to the twelfth centuries documented their local investigations into reported regional phenomena. During the Song dynasty, records of these investigations included notebooks, travel accounts, and inventories of things.[28] These three genres, owing to their item-by-item style and broad coverage of subject matter, allowed more room to account for new knowledge and, accordingly, became a popular written platform through which Song authors recorded their multifarious findings. Entries in these works unmistakably manifested their authors' reliance on the empirical strategy in their accounts of regional phenomena.[29] Those works resembled *Elucidating the Meaning* to the extent that they combined reliance on empirical investigation with erudition. Like Kou Zongshi, the authors in these cases compared their empirical findings meticulously with previously published textual records.[30]

The late ninth century, at the dusk of the Tang dynasty, witnessed a trend in which scholar-officials documented their empirical verifications of what they had previously read and heard about the Lingnan region (literally, "south of the Ling ranges") in far southern China. Observers have attributed this trend to the Tang people's curiosity about the far south, a remote and exotic region where the climate, creatures, local products, and customs all diverged from what was found in the central plains.[31] Although the term already appears in sources before the Tang dynasty, Lingnan officially became the name of one of ten administrative circuits that the Tang court established in 627.[32] The Lingnan circuit encompassed present-day Fujian, Guangdong, Hainan Island, most of Guangxi, the southeastern part of Yunnan, and the northern part of Vietnam. In the early Tianbao era (742–756), Fu and Zhang Prefectures (both in Fujian) were removed.[33] This change in effect defined the concept of Lingnan in later eras of imperial China. From that point on, "Lingnan" (or "Lingbiao" or "Liangwai") as a term referred mainly to Chinese territory that was located south of the Nanling Mountains (also known as the Wuling Mountains), a major mountain range in southern China that separates the Pearl River Basin from the Yangzi Valley.[34]

The emblem of this late Tang trend is Duan Gonglu's *Records of the Land of Northward-Facing Doors* (Beihu lu, hereafter *Northward-Facing Doors*). The term "northward-facing doors" (*beihu*) comes from an ancient dictionary,

Approaching Correctness (Erya, ca. 3rd century BCE), which used it in reference to the most remote region in the south.[35] Scholars between the Han and Qing dynasties had proposed various explanations as to why the region was so named. The famous Tang scholar Yan Shigu (581–645), for instance, explained that the name referred to a regional phenomenon; that is, the area was so far south that the sun shone only on its northern slopes and the locals thereby built their houses with the front doors facing the north to catch the sunlight.[36] Accordingly, imperial authors often used the term "northward-facing doors" to refer to the far south of China.

Duan resided in Xiang Prefecture (in Hubei) early in the Xiantong era (860–874), moving southward and living in Lingnan between 869 and 874. During this period in Lingnan, Duan resided in Gaoliang (in present-day Gaozhou city, Guangdong) in 869. He returned to Gaoliang from Pan Prefecture (Maoming city in Guangdong) in 870 and moved to the South Sea in 871. Sometime between 874 and 876, he met the regional military governor of the Lingnan East Circuit, Wei He, and very likely worked for him for a while. Duan's known post was defender of Wannian County under the jurisdiction of the Tang capital Chang'an (in Shaanxi).[37] In the extant three-*juan* edition of *Northward-Facing Doors*, nine out of fifty-two entries (17%) use the empirical strategy.[38] When accounting for the strategy, Duan often referred to himself as "Gonglu," "I" (*yu*), and "I, in my state of ignorance" (*yu*).

The written format of *Northward-Facing Doors* was devoted to a given region and presented a wide range of subject matter (including indigenous creatures, artifacts, disorders, and customs) in an item-by-item style, but it did not further systemize the subject matter by tying obvious threads together. These features can also be found in a literary corpus that emerged during the late Eastern Han era (25–220). That literature shared a common mark insofar as all of the works' titles included the phrase "records of exceptional things" (*yiwu zhi*). This body of work comes down to us only in the form of fragmented entries that were cited in later Six Dynasties, Tang, and Song works across a variety of genres, such as pharmacological collections, agricultural manuals, and "classified books" (*leishu*).[39] On the one hand, no empirical strategy is discernible in the extant fragmented entries of these works. On the other, some book titles in this literary corpus, such as *Records of Exceptional Things in Jiao Prefecture* (Jiaozhou yiwu zhi), suggest that their authors were devoted to recording exceptional occurrences in a specific region.[40] Regardless of their common features, Duan's strong emphasis on his empirical verification of

Lingnan-related topics distinguishes *Northward-Facing Doors* from earlier writings on regional features.

Duan verified claims through observations and inquiries. We see evidence of this practice in the entry on "*tong* rhinoceros" (*tongxi*). This entry began with anecdotes about rhinoceroses that Duan collated from five works, which included *Records of Exceptional Things in Southern Prefectures* (Nanzhou yiwu zhi). Following these anecdotes, Duan described the remarkable efficacy of rhinoceros horns when treating wounds pierced by poisonous plants, and he argued that "I additionally translated it from natives. This thing is not bogus." Duan then considered shells taken from live "hawksbill turtles" (*daimao*). Explaining their great efficacy when used to treat poisoning, he wrote "I, in my state of ignorance, had taken the shell to treat poison, and it immediately achieved the effect."[41]

Although he cited pharmacological collections in *Northward-Facing Doors*, Duan exerted little effort to challenge them; he primarily transcribed their records alongside other textual references. Only in one entry did he raise doubts about records in a pharmacological manual. In it, he questions whether the purpose of burning "owls" (*xiao*) was not to enjoy those birds' meat, an explanation that he cited from Chen Cangqi's *Collecting the Omissions,* but simply to kill them.[42] Duan provided no evidence in support of his alternative explanation.

The empirical strategy also appears in three other works that were written in the late Tang and early Five Dynasties (907–979) eras: *Miscellany of the Wilderness in Which I Was Positioned* (Touhuang zalu), by the regional inspector of Gao Prefecture (in Guangdong) in the early Dazhong era (847–860), Fang Qianli; *Records of Wind and Land of Guilin* (Guilin fengtu ji, 899), by the regional inspector of Rong Prefecture (in Guangxi), Mo Xiufu; and Liu Xun's *Recording the Extraordinary beyond the Ling Ranges* (Lingbiao luyi).[43] Notably, those three works, all of which involved the empirical strategy, attended primarily to affairs in Lingnan. Along with *Northward-Facing Doors*, they were classified under the bibliographical section of "historiographies" in standard histories but shared the same common characteristics of Song works that modern scholars have identified as notebooks. Those characteristics adopt an item-by-item presentation style; a less systematic format for the size, structure, and contents of the items; no clear thematic thread organizing or sequencing an array of the items; and a wide range of subject matter. To underscore these characteristics shared by these four late-Tang works and Song notebooks, I classified them as notebooks instead of as historiographies.

Duan Gonglu's family legacy presumably intensified his passion for verifying things and writing his verifications down. Duan Chengshi (ca. 800–863), who was presumably Duan Gonglu's uncle, composed the famous *Miscellaneous Morsels from Youyang* (Youyang zazu), which covers a broad range of topics, such as rituals, creatures, food, medicine, tales, architecture, and so forth.[44] It also shares an interest in the empirical strategy with *Northward-Facing Doors*. Duan Chengshi combined the experiences and verifications that he accumulated in various regions (including Shaanxi, Sichuan, Jiangsu, Zhejiang, and Jiangxi) along with firsthand information, hearsay, and textual sources, to compose *Miscellaneous Morsels*. He used the empirical strategy, for instance, in an entry in which he described his observations of ants in Chang'an during the Yuanhe era (806–820).[45] In another entry on "*tianniu* insects" (*tianniu chong*, presumably black beetles), he recalled that, in the summer in Chang'an, whenever the beetles appeared, it would rain; he said that he confirmed this phenomenon as many as seven times.[46]

The grand councilor Lu Xisheng (?–895) interpreted the rising visibility of the empirical strategy in *Northward-Facing Doors* as a counterbalance to the popularity of tales during that period, as shown in Lu's preface to it, according to which Duan Gonglu asked Lu to write the preface because Duan believed that Lu's having resided in Lingnan for years would have enabled him to "comprehensively examine facts that it [*Northward-Facing Doors*] recorded." This rationale indicates Duan's effort to vindicate the factuality of *Northward-Facing Doors*, especially considering that few authors in the Tang and Five Dynasties eras asked others to write prefaces for them.[47] Lu's appreciation of Duan's verification established the tone of his preface, which reads: "[Duan Gonglu] did not end his book merely with what he heard and saw, but furthermore linked it with similar cases, cited evidence, and compared and verified it with extraordinary books and exceptional statements. It is indeed broad and trustworthy."[48] "Broadness" (*bo*), on my reading, recognizes the wide scope of textual references in *Northward-Facing Doors*.[49] "Trustworthiness" (*xin*) refers not only to Duan's hearing and seeing but also to his critical skills in citing textual evidence and verifying exceptional statements.

Lu concluded his preface by drawing a contrast between *Northward-Facing Doors* and tales (*xiaoshuo*, literally, "small talks"). Novels, which were popular in the Tang era, especially in Lu's and Duan's day, were tales that varied widely in length and covered a broad range of themes, such as gossip, lore, romance, supernatural beings, and remarkable events.[50] Despite their popularity, though, Lu in the preface complains that many of them were either absurd and ridiculous or entertaining and humorous, meant to provoke laughter and merriment. Apart from those two types of work, Lu said that other tales "slandered earlier worthies, causing the multitude to take them as a subject of gossip."[51]

Following this criticism, Lu drew a contrast: "This is the pervasive ailment of recent times. What you [Duan Gonglu] said has none of it. What *Northward-Facing Doors* recorded all can be examined and verified. It is an assistance of broad learning of things; how could it be merely talking materials?"[52] Lu highlighted the scholarly value of *Northward-Facing Doors* by contrasting it with contemporary novels that in his opinion lacked factuality and were therefore suited only for gossip. Lu also described *Northward-Facing Doors* as a contribution to the "broad learning of things" (*bowu*).[53]

The contrast shows that Lu, as a historical actor, consciously distinguished literary genres written for entertainment purposes from those that were intended to convey knowledge. The latter could be called "epistemic genres," an analytic concept that the medical historian Gianna Pomata has developed.[54] Admittedly, Lu, like other historical actors in middle-period China, did not develop particular vocabularies to signify distinct epistemic genres. Nevertheless, his preface to *Northward-Facing Doors*, especially his description of the treatise's empirical features and the contrast between it and other literary genres that were intended primarily for amusement, indicates his awareness and appreciation of epistemic genres, in particular texts based on thorough empirical investigation. It is a pity that Lu did not further elaborate on what he meant by referring to this "broad learning of things," such as which texts would fall under this rubric and how the genre developed in the Tang era.

Lu Xisheng's comments on *Northward-Facing Doors* here are reminiscent of the Southern Song appreciation of a notebook's reliability and of the critical skills through which such reliability is achieved. Existing scholarship has found that it was not until the twelfth century that notebook authors began to value reliability and critical skills for their own sake; before then, the "dominant rhetoric for evaluating the credibility of a *biji* was to compare it to official histories."[55] Lu's preface demonstrated, however, the fledging consciousness of the idea of evaluating the credibility of notebook-style writing outside the framework of the historiographical tradition, hinting at the heightened value of the reliability and critical skills of notebooks since the late ninth century.

CONTINUITY AND CHANGE IN THE SONG ERA

From the tenth to the twelfth century, the trend toward applying the empirical strategy to support authors' statements about regional phenomena continued and intensified, appearing in notebooks and travel accounts.

Notebooks applying empirical strategy began to cover a wider range of topics than those in the late Tang era. This broader knowledge base can be seen in their titles, which were no longer devoted to specific regions. A case in point is *Trifling Talks from Northern Dreams* (Beimeng suoyan, hereafter *Northern Dreams*) by Sun Guangxian (?–968). Sun came from Ling Prefecture (in Sichuan), took refuge in Jingnan (in Hubei), worked for its ruler sometime between 926 and 963, and became a regional inspector in Huang Prefecture (in Hubei) after 963.

An existing but fragmented entry of *Northern Dreams* offers evidence of Sun's use of the empirical strategy. He began with a citation drawn from Chen Cangqi's *Collecting the Omissions*.[56] It said that *shafu* (literally, "captured by sand") was called *fuyu* by the Shu people, and when incorporated into pillows, it could render husbands and wives more loving of each other. Sun then described the process through which he verified this record. While traveling in Chengdu (in Sichuan), he became familiar with a "Mountain Man Lee" (Li *shanren*), who sold herbs and drugs. He often saw young men in Chengdu visiting Lee joyfully and paying him a "good price." Sun asked Lee what they were paying for. "Seduction drugs" (*meiyao*), Lee replied. Sun thereupon requested one of these drugs and discovered that it was the substance "captured by sand." Sun concluded his description of the process by noting that "what Chen said is trustworthy and not empty words." This entry was soon transcribed into an encyclopedia that the Song court compiled between 977 and 978, *Extensive Accounts of the Reign of Great Peace* (Taiping guangji).[57]

No notebook better reflects the continuing trend in the Northern Song than Shen Kuo's *Brush Talks* series.[58] In it, which modern scholars have analyzed in detail, Shen often recorded his hands-on experience in verifying topics ranging from musicology to astronomy to medicine to local affairs. He accounted for his witnessing of the appearance of the "thunder ax" in Sui Prefecture (in Hubei), his observations of "rainbow drinking water" on his diplomatic mission to the Liao (the northern neighbor of the Song), and his encounter with an "alligator" in Fujian.[59] In an entry about "black ghosts" (*wugui*), for instance, he wrote down what he witnessed to confirm the existence of a local custom about which he had once read.[60] Shen's introduction to this custom started with a poem written by the preeminent poet Du Fu (712–770), which reads, "Every household raises black ghosts, at every meal they eat yellow fishes." The Song scholar Liu Ke claimed that, according to *The Kui Prefecture Map Guide* (Kuizhou tujing), locals called fishing cormorants "black ghosts" and every household in the Shu area living next to water raised them, tying snares to the birds' necks and commanding them to fish in rivers. Once a cormorant caught a fish, the fishers brought the bird back in its upside-down position so as to let it spit the fish up. Shen recalled that, when staying there, he saw households that raised cormorants to fish, saying, "Liu Ke's words are trustworthy."[61]

Another eleventh-century notebook reflecting this empirical trend is *Mingdao's Miscellany* (Mingdao zazhi) by Zhang Lei (1054–1114, *jinshi* 1073), which was written between 1096 and 1102. A considerable number of entries in *Mingdao's Miscellany* apply the empirical strategy to discuss various topics, such as diet, ways of making brushes, local customs, trips, and so forth. An entry on Huang Prefecture (in Hubei) merits special attention, given that it argues against conventional wisdom in pharmacological collections, as *Elucidating the Meaning* did. Zhang, as a loyal follower of Su Shi, was demoted to Huang Prefecture between 1097 and 1098 when the New Policies faction, which was hostile to Su Shi, returned to power and resolved to stamp out the opposition. The entry on Huang Prefecture introduces multiple dimensions of the place, including its location, landscape, popularity, city walls, and customs; its residents' typical livelihoods and the vernacular accent; and products extracted from the mountains. At the very end of the entry, Zhang Lei mentioned pharmacological collections:

> Things of the insect and reptile category are mainly snakes. The one known as White Flower [a snake] cures wind-inducing disorders. Those that come from the neighboring Qi Prefecture are very expensive. Even when those from Huang Prefecture are dead, they have eyes that gleam and have been shown to cure disorders. The natives are able to catch them; one is sent as an annual tribute to the imperial treasury. The Huang people say this snake does not pursue its prey. It lies coiled in the grass and eats those things that come to it. Its curative powers are not quite what is said in pharmacological collections. When I was ill with "scabies" (*jiexian*), I ate three whole snakes and saw no effect.[62]

The quoted statement is strongly reminiscent of Kou Zongshi's entries in *Elucidating the Meaning*. Both entries are first-person narratives. The two authors did not adopt typical components in their introductions to medicinal substances. More importantly, both disagreed with pharmacological collections on the basis of their local experience, although Zhang Lei registered his challenge in a milder tone.

Regarding travel accounts, "Account of a Trip to the Stone Bell Mountain" (*Shizhongshan ji*) by Su Shi (1037–1101, *jinshi* 1057) is an example of using empirical strategy to buttress authors' opinions of regional phenomena. Modern scholarship has observed that Su was one of several eminent writers in the Northern Song era "who used travel records to advance particular arguments," which was a novel approach.[63] His account of Stone Bell Mountain indeed shares features with entries in *Elucidating the Meaning*.

Su Shi opens this travel account by expressing doubt about conventional explanations of the name "Stone Bell Mountain" proposed by two famous writers: Li Daoyuan (ca. 470–527) and Li Bo (fl. early 9th century). Li Daoyuan's *Commentary on the Classic of Waterways* (Shuijing zhu), Su stated, held that there was a deep pool next to the mountain, and that water in the pool tolled like bells when it struck rocks. Su noted that others had doubted Li Daoyuan's explanation, because even if one placed a bell into the water, there was no wind or waves that were strong enough to make it ring. Su recounted that Li Bo once found a pair of rocks along the bank of a pool and knocked them, finding their sound clanking. "I very much doubted it [Li Bo's claim]," Su commented. Su further pointed out that this claim could not explain why the mountain alone was named after a bell, given that the clanking sound made by rocks was supposed to be the same everywhere.

Su then noted that, in 1086, in the evening, when the moonlight was bright, he rode a small boat to the base of a steep precipice on Stone Bell Mountain with his son, Su Mai (1059–1119). They discovered rocky caves and fissures everywhere below the mountain. Any gentle waves that poured into the caves would knock the rocks and make sounds like gongs. When their boat on its return reached a point between two mountains, they saw a huge rock located in the middle of the channel. It was hollow in its center, with numerous apertures. When swallowed by or washed over by water and wind, the rock produced bangs and clanks that echoed the earlier sounds, as if musical bells were ringing. Su concluded his travel account as follows:

> Is it acceptable for someone who has not personally seen and heard something to have decided views on whether or not it exists? Li Daoyuan probably

saw and heard the same things I did, yet he did not describe them in detail. Scholar-officials have always been unwilling to take a small boat and moor it beneath the steep precipice at night. This is why they were unable to know the facts. Although fishers and boatmen who lived around Stone Bell Mountain knew about it, they were unable to describe it in writing. This is the reason that [the truth] has not been passed down through the generations. Imbeciles sought the answer by using axes to strike the rocks. Then they held that they had found out the fact of the matter. I thereupon made a record of these events to sign over Li Daoyuan's laconic explanation and Li Bo's imbecilic claim.[64]

The narrative structure of the record resembles some of Kou Zongshi's entries in *Elucidating the Meaning*, such as the one on fishing cormorants. The structure of such a record is first to indicate discrepancies in existing texts, then to present the author's personal verification, and finally to conclude with the author's comments on those texts.

In the account of Stone Bell Mountain and the above quotation in particular, Su Shi proposes a new model of qualification among scholar-officials. He advocated that they should see or hear things in person before drawing their conclusions; this compared unfavorably with the practices of Li Bo and those who were unwilling to conduct local investigations. Similar advocacy also appears in Kou Zongshi's criticism of Tao Hongjing. Su maintained that scholar-officials should, unlike Li Daoyuan, articulate their mode of verification, given that they had the capacity to write but others who knew the truth (such as the fishers and boatmen) did not. The same assessment of travel and personal investigation as an essential way of gaining knowledge appeared extensively in Song writings that immediately followed, including *Elucidating the Meaning*.[65]

This trend toward documenting authors' local investigations into purportedly regional phenomena continued well into the later Song period and proliferated in other written genres, such as local gazetteers.[66] Paralleling this trend, the number of notebooks produced after the mid-eleventh century increased similarly. Historians have considered this rising number a reflection of a new literati culture, which underlined the diversity and particularity of objects and affairs, contradicting the intellectual belief in one's capacity to understand relationships between Confucian classics, humans, and the cosmos in a systematic way.[67]

Notebooks constituted a prevalent written platform in which authors delivered their pharmacological knowledge in a relatively casual and informal style, as shown in abovementioned examples drawn from *Northern Dreams* and *Mingdao's Miscellany*. Shen Kuo in *Brush Talks* even devoted an entire chapter (*juan*) to medicinal substances, entitled "Discussion of Medicinals" (*Yaoyi*).[68] Like entries in *Elucidating the Meaning*, those in this chapter addressed a rich variety of topics concerning medicinal substances without following the conventional formats that were typical of pharmacological collections. The topics encompassed matching names with the substances in question, articulating rationales for choosing the seasons in which to collect substances, introducing prescription strategies for a drug, and arguing against previous or contemporary "incorrect" drug applications. *Brush Talks* itself encompassed a broad range of topics, reflecting Shen Kuo's interest in textual and experiential knowledge. The chapter "Discussion of Medicinals" manifests his familiarity with medical and pharmacological knowledge.[69]

The expanding presence of informal styles of conveying pharmacological knowledge from the late Tang to the Northern Song period helps to explain Kou Zongshi's confidence in writing up a considerable number of entries in an informal style (as many as 470) and even in collecting those entries into an independent book.

To be sure, Kou did not adduce every abovementioned text in *Elucidating the Meaning*. Nevertheless, the wide array of textual sources cited and collated in *Elucidating the Meaning* marks him as an educated man who was familiar with a considerable number of literary works produced before and during the Song dynasty. Those textual sources included *Approaching Correctness*, poems by famous Tang writers (including Li Bai [701–762], Du Fu [712–770], Han Yu [768–824], Bai Juyi [772–846], and Du Mu [803–852]), and renowned Buddhist travel accounts such as *Accounts of the Western Regions During the Great Tang* (Datang xiyuji, 646), *Miscellaneous Morsels from Youyang*, and an "inventory of things" written by Cai Xiang (1012–1067, *jinshi* 1030) and titled *Inventories of Lychee* (Lizhi pu).[70]

Of the abovementioned notebooks and travel accounts, Shen Kuo's *Brush Talks* is an important source for *Elucidating the Meaning*. On the one hand, Kou did not cite *Brush Talks* directly. On the other, six of Kou's entries contained sentences that were almost identical to those preserved in the "Discussion of Medicinals" chapter of *Brush Talks*.[71] Of those, fully half of the contexts in two entries bear striking similarities to items in *Brush Talks*.[72] Kou's use of *Brush Talks* without citing it as a reference is puzzling, considering that he mentioned Shen Kuo by name in other entries. Notwithstanding this unusual silence about a source, the inclusion of six entries renders *Brush Talks* the second most significant nonmedical textual source of *Elucidating the Meaning*, the first being *Monthly Ordinances* (Yueling), which is mentioned in eight entries. It is hard to explain Kou's unattributed use of *Brush Talks* given that he explicitly cites other contemporaneous writers' notebook-style works, such as *Inventories of Lychee*.

In addition to including the chapter "Discussion of Medicinals," *Brush Talks* bears other points of resemblance to *Elucidating the Meaning*. Argumentation permeates *Brush Talks*. In it, Shen Kuo displayed a strong commitment to accurately matching an object or affair with its lexical expression when accounting for textual and empirical testimony (such as observation) related to a phenomenon (such as the aforementioned entry on "black ghosts"), and presenting a penetrating understanding of an object, affair, or phenomenon. Like Kou Zongshi, Shen also mentioned the term "coherence" (*li*) in *Brush Talks* but showed little interest in endorsing it as omnipresent in everything across the world.[73]

The similarities between accounts of regional phenomena collected in notebooks, travel accounts, and *Elucidating the Meaning*—and the resemblance between it and *Brush Talks*—did not mean that those notebooks and travel accounts directly influenced the creation of *Elucidating the Meaning*. After all, there are too few surviving sources of information regarding Kou Zongshi to make it possible to reconstruct his intellectual inspiration with confidence. Instead, the similarities identify *Elucidating the Meaning* as part of a trend in which authors had, since the late ninth century, documented their local investigations into purported regional phenomena. Kou differed critically from those authors of notebooks and travel accounts, however, in the very act of submitting his work to the court.

EARNING STATE RECOGNITION

Kou Zongshi completed *Elucidating the Meaning* in 1116 and submitted it to the court that same year. Existing scholarship has attributed Kou's action to an edict commissioned in 1027. It required anyone who planned to print "individual collected works" (*wenji*) to submit them to the government; only after undergoing censorship would the collections be granted permission to be printed.[74] The scholarship also claims that Kou's status as an official and his use of *Elucidating the Meaning* to challenge the Song court–compiled pharmacological texts together prompted him to submit his work to the court as a response to the edict.[75] However, this claim does not take into account that the genres subject to the edict were literary collections, not medical treatises. Therefore, it cannot fully explain Kou's submission.

A more direct impetus for Kou's submission was a set of policies that elevated the status of medicine in Huizong's reign. More importantly, it may have been due to his aspirations to ascend the bureaucratic ladder by submitting to the court a putatively trustworthy pharmacological collection that supplemented and rectified earlier ones. This aspiration can be observed both in Kou's awareness of the Song government's support of medical publication and education and also in his assertive declaration regarding how his work modified *Jiayou Materia Medica* and *Illustrated Materia Medica*; both appear in the first chapter of *Elucidating the Meaning*.[76]

Kou began the first chapter by drawing an analogy between sages and Northern Song emperors who advocated for medicine. Kou placed the Song government's medical policies in the context of the sages' benevolence and desire to relieve the public of suffering. Kou first elaborated on how sages "regretted" (*min*) that the rest of humankind continuously suffered from disorders that were followed by death, offering medications and techniques designed to protect and preserve life. "This is why," Kou declared, "the state compiled *The Imperial Grace Formulary*, edited *Basic Questions*, corrected pharmacological collections again, and additionally prepared *Illustrated Materia Medica*. Works such as Zhang Ji's *Treatise on Cold Damage, Essential Formulas, Golden Chest*, and the *Imperial Library Formulary* are excellent and preserved in libraries."[77] The project of "correcting pharmacological collections again" refers to *Jiayou Materia Medica*, which was compiled to correct errors in *Kaibao Materia Medica*, which the early Song court had composed. The long list of government-commissioned medical treatises attests to Kou's awareness of the Song state's sponsorship of medical publications.

Kou continued by reviewing the medical education reforms implemented by Huizong's government. He remarked, "Nowadays, physicians under the heavens are selected by examination. Official titles and government offices are bestowed upon them. They are individually assigned to function-specific sections."[78] This quotation refers to policies supporting a larger project in which Huizong's government endeavored to raise the status of medicine and medical officials.[79] At the heart of this effort lay the reformation and expansion of medical education. The project began in 1103, when the Medical Academy (Yixue) was established under the Directorate of Education, a prestigious institution.[80] Other such academies were soon established in other cities. They were educational institutions operated by local and central governments to train well-educated men to become medical officials in government service.[81] By raising the status of medicine, Huizong's government aimed to attract students already educated in Confucian classics to attend medical academies, thus producing, in its term, "scholar-physicians" (*ruyi*, or literati physicians).[82] Between 1103 and 1120, polices pertinent to Kou's claim about physicians include those issued in 1115 that ordered the establishment of a medical academy in every prefecture and county and reregulated the examinations that determined the placement of students in such academies.[83] These policies, in Kou's words, were all attributed to "noble rulers who possess consummate wisdom and the greatest virtue."[84] The abolition of the Medical Academy in the capital in 1120 marked the diminishment of the endeavor.[85]

Two other policies that Kou Zongshi did not mention but were relevant to his submission of *Elucidating the Meaning* merit our attention here. One concerns the government's reaction when receiving unsolicited medical treatises during Huizong's reign. In 1111, Zhu Gong (fl. ca. 11th century, *jinshi* 1088?), a retired civil official, sent his son to submit his formulary, *One Hundred Questions on Cold Damage* (Shanghan baiwen), to the court.[86] Its objective was to explicate the *Treatise on Cold Damage*. Like *Jiayou Materia Medica*, *The Treatise on Cold Damage* was printed by the court in the eleventh century and served as a textbook for students in medical academies under Huizong's reign. Zhu perfectly fit the government's policy of recruiting scholar-physicians to participate in medical academies. The court named Zhu the "erudite master of the medical academy" (*yixue boshi*) in 1114. Zhu's return to officialdom (even though as a medical official) set the precedent for submitting medical treatises as a means of climbing the bureaucratic ladder.[87] This was an important element in the backdrop to Kou's submission of *Elucidating the Meaning*.

Another policy that was relevant to Kou's submission involved an "imperially brushed" (*yubi*) edict in 1114 that allowed individuals to "report and submit" "marvelous medical formulas and decent healing techniques" (*qifang shanshu*) to officials in their prefectures so as to pass them on to the court.[88] An imperially brushed directive was directly issued by the emperor to the agencies involved. During Huizong's reign, such directives were not only issued more frequently than in earlier Song courts, but they were also written in "slender gold" (*shoujin*), a distinctive style of calligraphy created by Huizong. The higher frequency of directives and the unique style of calligraphy helped extend and highlight the presence of the emperorship in the operation of government business.[89] The imperially brushed edict of 1114 manifested Huizong's determination to assemble remedies and healing techniques across China as comprehensively as possible. Although pharmacological collections did not directly fall within the parameter of the texts to be assembled, the edict nevertheless reiterated the government's openness to receiving unsolicited medical works.

Returning to the first chapter in *Elucidating the Meaning*, after praising medical policies under earlier Song emperors and Huizong, Kou Zongshi took up critiquing the compliers of *Jiayou Materia Medica* and *Illustrated Materia Medica*. The weight of Kou's criticism was proportional to the significance of these titles in Song medical education. The Song court had treated the compilation of the two pharmacological encyclopedias seriously, having issued an edict in 1058 calling for the collection of information regarding medicinal substances that originated across and beyond China. The edict ordered each circuit, prefecture, and district not only to report the locations where their indigenous medicinal substances originated but also to submit information on and illustrations of them. With respect to medicinal substances that originated in foreign lands, it was up to local governors to assign someone to interview merchants in official border markets and seaborne traders and to submit one or two specimens of each foreign substance to the capital. On the basis of all of the information, illustrations, and specimens collected from localities at great effort, *Jiayou Materia Medica* and *Illustrated Materia Medica* were compiled.[90] The former then served as the textbook for all students in medical academies from as early as 1103.[91] The government's expansion of medical education from the capital across the prefectures in 1115 rapidly multiplied the number of its readers.

In spite of the thorough process through which *Jiayou Materia Medica* and *Illustrated Materia Medica* were compiled, Kou Zongshi harshly criticized them. He commented that the compilers of the two pharmacological encyclopedias primarily expressed their personal opinions and failed to consult other authors or compare their own work with theirs; as a result, medical "learners" (*xuezhe*) were not able to consult the two sources "without confusion" (*wuhuo*).[92]

Kou then shifted the narrative focus to the advantages of his own work over medical learning:

> I have now examined the statements of numerous authors and compared them with the facts. With regard to statements that do not elaborate the coherence

[*jueli*] of a healing substance, I have elucidated them to establish that they meet the criteria of coherence, as in the case of [1] soil made of eastward walls, [2] water not flowing downward, and [3] winter ashes. With regard to those where meanings are hidden and evasive and are not easily discerned, I have expanded on them to expose their conditions [*qing*], as in the case of [4] water passing beneath chrysanthemum flowers that becomes aromatic and in the case of [5] the mole's essence of urine that drops onto the earth and thereby engenders offspring. With regard to those which are mistaken and omitted in characters and manuscripts, I have proven this by means of clarifying their meanings, as in the case of [6] jade spring water and [7] stone honey. As far as the name of some drugs that had been changed to avoid mentioning the names of emperors are concerned, I have traced them back to the original source to preserve their names, as in the case of [8] yam [*shanyao*, literally, "mountain drugs"], whose character falls under a taboo of the present dynasty; during the Tang period, the name of Emperor Daizong was banned. Thereby I have rendered the right and wrong to become one; therapies have a basis; in the moment when medical learners consulted and applied pharmacological collections, they are enlightened without confusion.[93]

By listing four types of corrections to the *Jiayou Materia Medica* textbook, and by helping medical students consult pharmacological collections without confusion, Kou demonstrated the potential and pragmatic usefulness of his dedication to expanding government-sponsored medical education in his day. He concluded the first section of the first chapter with a declaration that the creation of *Elucidating the Meaning* was offered to "match our sage dynasty's virtue of loving life."

It is noteworthy that, in the proceeding quotation, Kou offers no novel term or expression to characterize his findings that he gained through his empirical investigations. Instead, he invested ink to describe his corrections to *Jiayou Materia Medica* and *Illustrated Materia Medica*. The descriptive nature of Kou's view of empirical knowledge echoed Shen Kuo's rich description of his findings in *Brush Talks*. The high proportion of entries using the empirical strategy occupy the eight entry examples in this quotation. Of these, two refer to entries employing the empirical strategy (the fourth and sixth examples). This attests to Kou's emphasis on his empirical verification.

After advertising the advantages of his *Elucidating the Meaning*, Kou declared that the classifications of drug entries in his work all followed *Jiayou*

Materia Medica and *Illustrated Materia Medica*.[94] He did not further explain the rationale for duplicating the classifications. One advantage of the duplication may be that it allowed medical learners to conveniently compare differences between drug entries in *Elucidating the Meaning* and those in the two Song court–compiled pharmacological encyclopedias.

Kou submitted *Elucidating the Meaning* to the Department of State Affairs (Shangshu Sheng) in 1116. The central government soon reviewed it. The manual was then sent to the Imperial Medical Academy (Taiyi Xue). The erudite master there, Li Kang, examined it, commenting that *Elucidating the Meaning* "is indeed a book whose author studied hard. Its meaning could be adopted." In February 1117, an imperial decree ordered the promotion of Kou Zongshi to the next higher official rank and assigned him an additional administrative task: examining the quality and authenticity of medicinal substances purchased by the central government, at the Institute for Collecting and Purchasing Drugs (Shoumai Yaocaisuo), an institution established in Kaifeng during the Chongning reign (1102–1106).[95] The new assignment moved Kou from the remote Li Prefecture to the prosperous Song capital. Li Kang's comments and Kou's new administrative assignment both indicate the Song court's recognition of the pharmacological value of *Elucidating the Meaning* and Kou's expertise in pharmacology.

State recognition was, nonetheless, far from demonstrating that Huizong's government aimed to advocate for the application of the empirical strategy in medical treatises. In fact, the government paid much more attention to a pharmacological encyclopedia that differed considerably from *Elucidating the Meaning*. It relied heavily on textual testimony and lacked argumentation. This heightened attention may imply that the government (or Huizong) preferred pharmacological collections based on textual testimony over those based on the empirical strategy. The original version of that encyclopedia was titled *Materia Medica Validated and Classified from the Classics and Histories for Emergency Preparedness* (Jingshi zhenglei beiji bencao, hereafter *Validated and Classified*). Its author, Tang Shenwei, was a famous physician in Sichuan and compiled his encyclopedia sometime between 1080 and 1094. Its aim was to revise *Jiayou Materia Medica* and *Illustrated Materia Medica*, the same objective as that of *Elucidating the Meaning*. As a renowned physician with numerous clients, Tang was assumed to have accumulated a vast storehouse of pharmacological knowledge from his healing encounters. In contrast, however, to Kou Zongshi, who documented his empirical investigations and medical cases, Tang rested

70 CHAPTER TWO

the knowledge claims in his work predominantly on textual evidence, as noted in the title of his encyclopedia.

The scope of Tang's textual references actually went far beyond classics and historiographies, extending to Daoist and Buddhist works, medical genres, and literary works, including as many as 220 titles.[96] The sheer number and wide range of the references are owed in part to Tang's "reimbursement" from his literate patients. In exchange for his medical services, Tang requested that they give him not money but pieces of writing that contained information about medical formulas or medicinal substances. It is likely that these pieces formed the main body of Tang's textual references.[97]

In addition to citing textual references as its central persuasion strategy, the information-management style in *Validated and Classified* likewise differs markedly from *Elucidating the Meaning*. Entries in *Validated and Classified* perfectly follow the typical format of introducing medicinal substances by referring to their flavors, qualities, main indications, and so forth. When juxtaposing separate textual sources under a given item, Tang rarely judged which sources were more accurate. This reluctance to judge indicates that he did not aim to provide accurate pharmacological information about individual medicinal substances. The absence of argumentation in *Validated and Classified* meanwhile obscures the presence and epistemic authority of Tang as its author. All of these features—preferred persuasion strategies, the information-management style, the attention to accuracy, and the visibility of authors' epistemic authority—contrast starkly with *Elucidating the Meaning*.

Later, Song officials and the court edited and expanded Tang's work. Ai Sheng (fl. 11th century), a "defender of the subprefecture" (*xianwei*) in Renhe County in Hang Prefecture (in Hangzhou city), noticed Tang's work and expanded on it by adding Chen Cheng's *Expanded Divine Farmer's Materia Medica and Illustrated Materia Medica*. Ai entitled this extended version *Materia Medica Validated and Classified from the Classics and Histories of the Daguan Reign* (Jingshi zhenglei daguan bencao, hereafter *Daguan Materia Medica*), printing it in 1108.[98] Eight years later, Huizong commissioned his favorite medical official, Cao Xiaozhong, to edit *Daguan Materia Medica*.[99] Cao accomplished the editing project in one month and submitted the book in 1116 under a new title, *Materia Medica Validated and Classified from the Classics and Histories for Practices, Newly Edited in the Zhenghe Reign* (Zhenghe xinxiu jingshi zhenglei beiyong bencao, hereafter *Zhenghe Materia Medica*). The editing project that involved *Zhenghe Materia Medica* suggested greater imperial appreciation of this pharmacological work than of *Elucidating the Meaning*. The Song empire fell in 1127 to its northern invaders, the Jurchen, who confiscated almost all the woodblocks with which books that were stored in the court were printed, in all likelihood including those for *Zhenghe Materia Medica*, which thereby did not stand a chance of being printed or circulating in the newly reconstituted Southern Song China.

For its part, *Elucidating the Meaning* was printed at least four times during the Southern Song era. The Fiscal Commission in Longxing Fu (in Nanchang) printed it in 1185, revising and reprinting it in 1195.[100] A private publisher in Fujian also printed *Elucidating the Meaning*, presumably in pursuit of financial gain.[101] The commercial publisher in Jianyang (in northern Fujian), "Yu Yanguo from the Hall of Encouraging Scholarly Worthies" (Yu Yanguo Lixian Tang, hereafter Yu Yanguo), integrated *Elucidating the Meaning* with *Daguan Materia Medica*, titling the new version *Newly Compiled and Edited Materia Medica with Illustrations and Commentaries* (Xinbian zhenglei tuzhu bencao) and printing it sometime between 1208 and 1241.[102] (Jianyang, by the way, had been one of the most significant centers of printing and the book trade in imperial China since the Song dynasty.[103]) Yu Yanguo abridged the contents of the two pharmacological texts and inserted the contents of drug entries from *Elucidating the Meaning* into corresponding drug entries in *Daguan Materia Medica*. This mode of integration renders *Elucidating the Meaning* one of many layers of commentaries involving drug entries in *Daguan Materia Medica* (fig. 2). This combined and abbreviated version not only allowed readers to consult the two texts at once but also made it more affordable when compared with the cost of purchasing complete versions of both *Elucidating the Meaning* and *Daguan Materia Medica*. These advantages may have facilitated sales of this version, subsequently expanding the circulation of *Elucidating the Meaning*.

DEPARTING FROM HIS PREDECESSORS, Kou Zongshi spurned typical formats for introducing medicinal substances that were established in pharmacological collections. Instead, he devoted many entries to argumentation, incorporating his medical cases and local investigations into *Elucidating the Meaning*. These features of his work bear similarities to some notebooks from the late Tang period and travel accounts under the Song. Beginning in the late ninth century, a growing number of scholar-officials began documenting their own investigations into regional phenomena about which they had read or heard, including information regarding medicinal substances. This intellectual legacy of the late

72   CHAPTER TWO

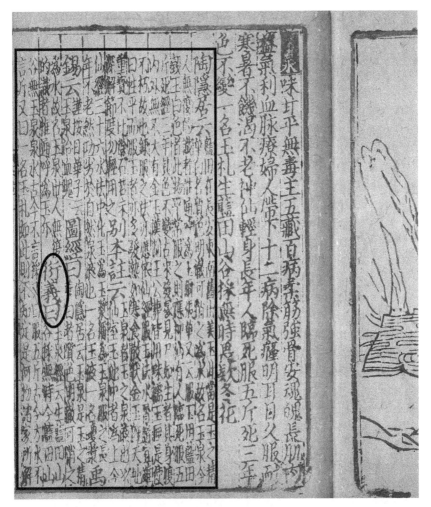

FIG. 2. Entry on jade spring in *Newly Compiled and Edited Materia Medica with Illustrations and Commentaries,* in an edition printed in the Yuan dynasty (1271–1368). The entry begins on the right-hand side with an illustration of jade spring water and four columns of large characters that describe its flavor, degree of heat, poison or potency (*du*) status, medical uses, locations, and collection seasons. The larger boxed section to the left contains commentaries on jade spring water drawn from pharmacological texts completed between the fifth and twelfth centuries. The circle highlights three large characters that mean "*Elucidating the Meaning* says" (Yanyi yue). The text in small characters following the circle is an extract from *Elucidating the Meaning*'s entry on jade spring water. Courtesy of the Institute of History and Philology, Academia Sinica, Taipei, Taiwan.

Tang and Five Dynasties eras survived into the Song era and further thrived. By the late eleventh century, authors' investigations alone provided sufficient support for their criticism of conventional understandings of certain regional phenomena. Their enhanced evidential value that this reflects appeared in both notebooks and travel accounts from the Song era. Meanwhile, the rising number of notebook-style writings since the mid-eleventh century meant that conveying knowledge in such informal styles became an increasingly acceptable option. This trend—the rising persuasive power of local investigations and the greater acceptability of informality—laid the foundation not only of Kou's reliance on empirical strategy but also of his confidence in criticizing court-commissioned pharmacological encyclopedias and submitting *Elucidating the Meaning* to Huizong's government. Findings yielded by Kou's method of empirical verification served as supporting evidence of the improvement that his work brought to pharmacological knowledge. After submitting his work, Kou received an administrative assignment in the capital, reflecting state recognition of his efforts.

Many Southern Song literary and medical works cited and mentioned *Elucidating the Meaning*. The first formulary devoted to treating women, *Comprehensive Good Medical Formulas for Women* (Furen daquan liangfang, 1237), records the medical case and formula for lamb soup that opens this chapter.[104] Authors of Southern Song notebooks, when discussing medicinal substances and plants, often drew on entries from *Elucidating the Meaning*.[105] The famous Song-dynasty bibliographer Chen Zhensun, in his bibliographical treatise *Zhizhai's Annotated Catalog*, openly praises the "evidence drawing, discernment, and validation" in *Elucidating the Meaning* and argues that it "richly deserved to be read and adopted." In contrast, Chen commented unfavorably on *Edited Materia Medica in the Shaoxing Regime* (Shaoxing jiaoding bencao, 1159), a pharmacological encyclopedia that the Southern Song court compiled. Chen said that its language was vulgar and its statements were rather commonplace.[106] This contrast exemplifies Southern Song authors' approval of *Elucidating the Meaning*.

The Song development of documenting contemporary experience into pharmacological collections furthermore enhances our understanding of the long-term trajectory of the empirical strategy in this genre, helping us to identify two remarkable differences that characterized the application of this persuasion strategy between the Song and early Qing periods. The first is the growing frequency of names of ordinary people who contributed their materia medica knowledge to a pharmacological collection author. The Tang and Song authors discussed in this chapter did not record names of the people they asked about medicinal substances. "Local folks" are the only title the informants enjoyed. In contrast, Zhao Xuemin (fl. 1753–1803), a sojourning private secretary, in his *Supplement to Systematic Materia Medica* (Bencao gangmu shiyi), recorded names of persons in lowbrow circles from whom he learned about medicinal substances.[107] The second feature is the wider geographical scope of information and material exchange via letters between pharmacological collection authors staying and traveling across the Qing empire and their informants. Although Song literati often exchanged goods and gifts via letters, they rarely used them as means of gaining new pharmacological information. Instead, as shown in this chapter, the Song authors preferred "field study."

Interestingly, although Shen Kuo and Kou Zhongshi had included ample medical cases in their treatises, the civil official and physician Xu Shuwei, in the mid-twelfth century, still claimed his treatise as the pioneering formulary appending medical formulas to cases. The claim and Xu's treatise are the subject of the next chapter.

THREE Demonstration of Medical Virtuosity

Someone had contracted cold damage disorder. His body felt hot, his eyes were painful, his nose was dry, he could not lie down, he was constipated.... These symptoms had lasted several days. One evening, he also began to sweat. I said: "Quickly use the Major Bupleurum Decoction [Da Chaihu Tang] to drain him downward." The assembled physicians were shocked, remarking: "When a patient experiences spontaneous sweating due to disorders of the Yang Brightness tract, it means that his body's "refined fluids" [*jinye*] have already drained. The method of treatment must be to apply a honey enema. What made you decide to use rhubarb [*dahuang*] for this patient?" I said: "You only know to play it safe. Using Major Bupleurum Decoction is one of Zhang Zhongjing's miraculous treatments that has not been transmitted. How could you fine gentlemen have known about it?" I insisted that this treatment was the correct one. Eventually, I administered the Major Bupleurum Decoction. After two doses, the patient was cured.

—Xu Shuwei, *Puji benshifang*, 8.143

THIS CASE NARRATIVE is drawn from *The Widely Benefiting Formulary with Explanatory Historical Contexts* (Puji benshifang, hereafter *The Formulary with Explanatory Historical Contexts*). Its author, the civil official and physician Xu Shuwei (1080–1154), completed the formulary and printed it late in life. Xu's case narratives, including the one above, differ remarkably from the Song ones we have encountered in the preceding two chapters. As we saw in chapter 1, Shen Kuo in *Good Formulas* was never ashamed to express his uncertainty about which are the best remedies to apply in particular cases. In contrast, Xu's case narrative not only exhibits strong confidence in the recommended therapy but also includes an attempt to justify its use. Xu does not shy away from acknowledging his debates with rival healers or his interest in competing with them for patient patronage, a scenario that is absent from Kou Zongshi's *Elucidating the Meaning,* the principal source analyzed in the preceding chapter. These features of Xu's case narrative—his high confidence in the treatment, his attempt to justify its use, and the representation of competition between physicians for patient patronage—collectively render this formulary distinct from medical treatises completed before and even in Xu's day. Rather, this early twelfth-century formulary looks more like the "medical case statements" (*yi'an*) that surfaced in the sixteenth century.

What factors inspired Xu Shuwei to compose this formulary that is seemingly ahead of its time? What did Xu seek to achieve by collecting his cases in a formulary?

XU SHUWEI'S LIFE AND HIS OEUVRE

Xu Shuwei practiced medicine as a physician and remained an examination candidate for several decades. At the age of fifty-two, he finally passed the civil service examination and hence became a civil official—he was a member of the ruling class. His life and career were so unique for the Song dynasty that he become something of a celebrity.

Song sources offer several accounts to explain why Xu practiced medicine. The variety of these accounts indicate his fame, suggesting that his life drew widespread attention.[1] Xu himself attributed his vocation to his parents' death when he was a child.[2] When he was eleven years old, his father and mother died from successive illnesses within a hundred days of one another. After growing up, Xu studied medicine diligently and became a physician. Hong Mai (1123–1202) offered an alternative version in his *Record of the Listener* (Yijian zhi), one of the most popular and widely disseminated notebook series in the Southern Song era. Hong declared that Xu chose to become a physician because saving lives enabled him to accumulate good karma and thereby helped him to pass competitive civil service examinations.[3] Xu indeed attempted the examinations several times, although we do not know how many. These examinations typically were administered every three years, but it seems that for several decades, Xu aspired to but failed to pass them.

Xu was not the first member of the elite to master the Confucian classics and go on to earn a living by healing the sick. Since at least the sixth century, some members of the classically educated elite staked their claim to fame or their livelihoods on medicine. Treating their parents' (usually their mothers') disorders constituted the primary motivation for learning and later comprehending the art of healing.[4] The ranks of the classically educated elite who chose medicine as an occupation grew conspicuously during the Song dynasty, especially after the eleventh century. Modern scholars have proposed several explanations for this phenomenon. One notes that the proposition that medicine was a knowledge domain worthy of the cultural elite was firmly established in this era. Another argues that public dissemination of medical literature enabled the literati to learn medicine from books.[5] The Song emperors' interest in and imperial patronage of medicine enhanced the esteem conferred on it as an occupation.[6] Facing the increasingly competitive civil service examination, many candidates who repeatedly failed saw practicing medicine as a physician as one of the next best options.[7] With this in mind, we can better understand how encouraging Xu's story would be for his educated Song fellows when he eventually passed the examination with flying colors late in his life. It was this late success that made him something of a legend.

The advantageous transport location of Xu's hometown, in Zhen Prefecture (in Jiangsu), helps to explain why he, as a local physician, was able to access texts that were instrumental in preparing for the civil service examination and in learning medicine. Zhen Prefecture is located at the confluence of the Grand Canal and the Yangzi River. Through the canal, goods that originated in the south were imported to the capital, Kaifeng, and other destinations in northern China. Through the Yangzi River transport network, goods were carried between eastern and western China. Located at the interface of these two central networks, Zhen Prefecture benefited from the transport of large volumes of materials and products across China.[8] Its location meant that, although his activity was mostly confined to the prefecture, Xu still had ample opportunity to access texts produced outside his home county. This circumstance informs our understanding of his success in the examination as well as of the variety of texts that he discussed in his works.

When Xu was forty-seven years old, the Jurchen Jin state besieged and sacked Kaifeng, ending the Northern Song dynasty. In the same year, the ninth son of Emperor Huizong ascended to the throne, establishing a successor state, known as the Southern Song. This regime waged war against the Jin, joining numerous and often violent engagements from 1127 to 1142 along the middle and lower reaches of the Yellow and Huai Rivers. Zhen Prefecture, which as indicated above was once a prosperous transfer port, now became a border region that was prone to Jin attacks. In addition to the Jin armies, gangs of bandits ravaged the prefecture as well; the leader of one gang of bandits, Zhang Yu, engaged in armed robbery and set fire to regions of it in 1128.[9] Following these ravages, "conglomeration diseases" (*jijia*) reached epidemic proportions. Xu Shuwei visited patients who were suffering from conglomeration diseases and healed 70 to 80 percent of them.[10]

While living in a turbulent time, Xu eventually passed the civil service examinations at the age of fifty-two and earned a fifth ranking nationally, a distinction of great honor. Varying versions of the story, according to which Xu passed the examinations with such distinction after saving countless lives, spread across the Southern Song region in medical treatises and notebooks. The popularity of anecdotes about Xu renders him one of the most frequently discussed medical writers of the era. Even the Southern Song gazetteer of Xu's home county, *Yizhen Gazetteer* (Yizhen zhi), documented Xu's life.[11]

Beyond anecdotes regarding Xu's performance on the examinations, extant Song sources say little about his official career. We know with certainty of only two particular positions that he held. Both were in the capital of the Southern Song state, Lin'an (in Hangzhou city). One position involved serving as a professor at the Lin'an Prefectural School in 1142, when the court assigned him to help with the metropolitan civil service examination.[12] He then became an official in the capital, but his specific title has not come down to us.[13] The other position was as the "academician of the Hanlin Academy" (*Hanlin xueshi*), an appointment reflecting great dignity, giving him responsibility for drafting imperial orders and edicts.[14] The latter appointment won Xu the posthumous title of Academician Xu (Xu Xueshi). Xu retired in an unknown year but apparently continued treating the sick.[15]

Xu Shuwei was a prolific author. He wrote at least seven medical treatises. As shown by their titles, most concerned cold damage disorders. "Cold damage" (*shanghan*), to be very brief, was a generic term used by medical authors in imperial China in reference to disorders that covered a wide variety of symptoms that were often ascribed to the invasion of the human body by seasonal or unseasonal cold qi. Some of the symptoms are reminiscent of what we know today as febrile illness. Of the seven treatises Xu wrote, he had already lost three by 1129 as casualties of military conflicts: *Diagrams about Zhongjing's Methods of Palpating the Pulse* (Zhongjing maifa sanshiliu tu), *Aid to the Treatise on Cold Damage* (Yi shanghan lun), and *Classified Differential Diagnosis* (Bianlei). Of the remaining four, one has been lost and is known only by its title: *Methods of Therapy in Eighty-One Sections* (Zhifa bashiyi pian). The other three have come down to us. Of those, Xu completed and printed *One Hundred Mnemonic Verses on Cold Damage Manifestations* (Shanghan baizheng ge) and *Subtleties of Cold Damage Revealed* (Shanghan fawei lun) around 1135.[16] The last one, *The Formulary with Explanatory Historical Contexts*, Xu finished and printed after 1143, when he was, in all likelihood, retired.[17] Because references to all seven titles appear in Xu's own writings, their authorship is certain.

Four other medical treatises were attributed to Xu Shuwei generations after his death. One was entitled *Instructions to Save Lives* (Huoren zhinan). According to the famous Southern Song scholar-official Lou Yue (1137–1213), this treatise concerned cold damage disorders.[18] The second was *Classified Examples of the Efficacy of Classics* (Jingxiao leili). The text has been lost, but its title suggests that it may have included healing case narratives as testimony to the efficacy of remedies that were applied according to medical classics. The third treatise was titled *Sequel to the Classified and Widely Benefiting Formulary with Explanatory Historical Contexts* (Leizheng puji benshifang xuji or Benshifang houji). Although it circulated in the thirteenth century, a Southern Song medical author doubted that Xu was its author.[19]

The fourth medical treatise attributed to Xu Shuwei after his death was *Ninety Discussions on Cold Damage Disorders* (Shanghan jiushi lun, hereafter *Ninety Discussions*). No surviving book attributed to Xu has attracted more scholarly attention than *Ninety Discussions*, which is distinguished from other Song medical treatises by its contents. Case narratives constituted its bulk, and those depict the healing practices of a single physician, Xu Shuwei. In contrast, formulas occupy a more central place than case narratives did in medical treatises completed in and before the Song dynasty. The case narratives collected in those treatises often come from both the authors' own medical cases and others' cases (as is true of Shen Kuo's *Good Formulas*). Some scholars hence regard *Ninety Discussions* as the forerunner of collections of medical case histories serving as a new genre in China.[20] Along the same line of thinking, Xu is the first physician to have written down and published a collection of his own medical case histories.

It is unlikely, however, that Xu was the author of *Ninety Discussions*. He never mentioned this treatise nor did anyone in the Southern Song talk about it. That *Ninety Discussions* was never documented in the Southern Song era is baffling, because it conflicts not only with Xu's fame but also with the popularity of his

Formulary with Explanatory Historical Contexts at the time. As a celebrity at the time, Xu was mentioned in numerous medical texts and notebooks; *The Formulary with Explanatory Historical Contexts* was widely cited and one of the most frequently printed medical treatises in the Song era. In contrast, the earliest fragments of *Ninety Discussions* appear in a fifteenth-century encyclopedic work, *Great Compendium of the Yongle Era*.[21] The Ming court completed this encyclopedia in 1408, some 250 years after Xu's death.

Comparing an identical case in *Ninety Discussions* and *The Formulary with Explanatory Historical Contexts* yields more solid evidence indicating that Xu is unlikely to have been the author of *Ninety Discussions*. In *The Formulary with Explanatory Historical Contexts*, there was a case in which Fan Yun (451–503) was subordinate to "Emperor Wu of the Liang dynasty" (Liang Wudi, personal name Xiao Yan, 464–549, r. 502–549). Fan contracted a cold damage disorder very suddenly, and he sought to be cured immediately so that he could attend a ceremony scheduled imminently that would showcase Xiao Yan's ruling power.[22] In *Ninety Discussions* the plot remained the same, but the figure "Emperor Wu of the Liang" was replaced by "Chen Baxian" (503–559, r. 557–559), who was Emperor Wu of the Chen dynasty.[23] This difference reveals serious gaps in literary and historical knowledge regarding the author of *Ninety Discussions* and Xu Shuwei.

Xu, in *The Formulary with Explanatory Historical Contexts*, explicitly documented that he drew the case from *History of the South* (Nanshi), a standard history completed in 659 that recorded political events occurring between 420 and 589.[24] As recorded there, Fan Yun had been friends with Xiao Yan long before the latter acceded to the throne. Xiao Yan, Fan Yun, and six other men of letters were collectively called "the eight companions of the prince of the Jingling" (*Jingling bayou*), an illustrious group in the world of literary men.[25] Their friendship explained why Fan was so eager to attend the ceremony held for Xiao. By replacing "Emperor Wu of the Liang dynasty" with "Chen Baxian," who flourished after Fan's death, the author of *Ninety Discussions* not only made an ahistorical mistake but also misunderstood Fan's career as recorded in the standard history, *History of the South*. Given that standard histories were texts that anyone in the Song era attempting to pass the civil service examinations were expected to learn, it would be surprising if Xu, who passed the examination and earned the "advanced scholar" degree, made such basic mistakes. I thus consider those mistakes important evidence indicating that the author of

Ninety Discussions was not Xu but rather someone with more limited literary and historical knowledge.

Recent scholarship also suggests that Xu was unlikely to have been the author of *Ninety Discussions*. Comparison of *Ninety Discussions* with two medical treatises that were certainly written by Xu—*Subtleties of Cold Damage Revealed* and *The Formulary with Explanatory Historical Contexts*—shows that the language used in *Ninety Discussions* was more colloquial than that in the other two treatises. For instance, *Ninety Discussions* mentions Emperor Wu of the Chen dynasty with his original name, Chen Baxian, whereas the other two treatises respectfully employ "Emperor Wu of the Liang." More importantly, some of prescription strategies included in *Ninety Discussions* directly contradict corresponding ones recommended in *Subtleties of Cold Damage Revealed*.[26] The colloquial language and the contradictions together make it more likely that the contents of *Ninety Discussions* were based on drafts of medical case records that Xu wrote. It would not be surprising to learn that healers in imperial China developed the habit of recording their successful cures for their own reference without leaking the records to others they did not know. The Western Han physician Chunyu Yi's "examination records" (*zhenji*) exemplify this practice. Xu may have kept a log of his clinical practices for his own purposes as well.

Rather than identifying Xu Shuwei as the author of *Ninety Discussions*, a more plausible scenario is that, based on the rough drafts of his medical case records, which Xu used to compose *Subtleties of Cold Damage Revealed* and *The Formulary with Explanatory Historical Contexts*, someone (perhaps disciples of Xu or his descendants) later compiled and edited those drafts into *Ninety Discussions* between the fall of the Southern Song dynasty and the fifteenth century. Considering the strong possibility that *Ninety Discussions* was not a Song-dynasty treatise, I do not analyze its case narratives in this study.

Unlike *Ninety Discussions*, which was apparently unknown in the Song context, *The Formulary with Explanatory Historical Contexts* received popular acclaim in the Song period. It was printed at least six times in Zhen Prefecture, Yong Prefecture (in Hunan), and Jianyang (in Fujian) in this era by various publishers, including Xu Shuwei himself, local officials positioned in Xu's home county, and private (or commercial) publishers.[27]

THE STRUCTURE OF XU SHUWEI'S CASE NARRATIVES

The extant version of *The Formulary with Explanatory Historical Contexts* consists of ten chapters covering remedies for a wide range of disorders. The chapters include some 362 remedies and 123 medical cases, including both Xu's and others' cases that he drew from previous texts or with which he was otherwise acquainted. Xu appended relevant case histories to a given medical formula. For instance, the narrative for the use of the Major Bupleurum Decoction, which we saw at the beginning of this chapter, follows the formula of the decoction. Case histories in *The Formulary with Explanatory Historical Contexts* vary in length. Some of them are as short as three sentences, whereas others extend over several paragraphs. In general, though, Xu's own were longer than others' and were often supplemented with detailed theoretical discussions. This formula-case-discussion trilogy format appears in other Song formularies as well.

Almost all of Xu's own case histories in *The Formulary with Explanatory Historical Contexts* follow the same general structure: Each one begins with information about a sick person's history, such as their surname, locale, occupation, and relationship to Xu. Each then describes the disorders in question, including symptoms, duration, and development over time, as well as the patient's relevant medical history, such as previous physicians' misdiagnoses and misprescribed treatments. A typical case ends with Xu's diagnosis and prescription, and the outcome for the sick person. In most cases, the patient followed Xu's advice and then recovered. Reporting successful outcomes helped to signal the reliability and enhance the credibility of the remedies Xu recorded. In some cases, a patient was too skeptical or bullheaded to accept Xu's prescription and subsequently died from their disorder. Their deaths ironically attest to Xu's amazing predictive skills.

In many cases, Xu included the rationale for his diagnosis and treatment in his replies to questions. Rival healers around sickbeds were not the only group raising such questions, as members of patients' households also did. Eager to see their loved ones recover quickly, those family members were opinionated and did not hesitate to replace healers they considered unsuccessful with others whom they regarded as more skillful.

After describing successful outcomes of his treatments, Xu sometimes cited or elaborated his analytic opinions of passages from other texts he regarded as relevant to specific disorders. Those passages came from both pre-Song and Song texts, as well as both medical and nonmedical texts, such as *The Book of*

DEMONSTRATION OF MEDICAL VIRTUOSITY   83

Songs (Shijing), *Essential Formulas,* and *Good Formulas.* The wide scope of the citations demonstrated Xu's familiarity with a great body of textual knowledge accumulated from the past but also extending into his day. In addition to commenting on other medical texts, Xu sometimes ended a case with a theoretical discussion, which encompassed a broad range of topics, from the origins of disorders in question to the rationale behind a diagnosis or prescription. These discussions often presented new medical ideas that Xu had developed over years of clinical practice.

Among the medical case histories included in *The Formulary with Explanatory Historical Contexts*, those involving treatment for cold damage, which are found in the eighth and ninth chapters, carry special weight. As shown in table 1, the ratio of Xu's medical cases to remedies is higher in most chapters than the ratio of other peoples' cases to remedies. The former reaches its peak in the eighth and ninth chapters. In contrast, the latter in these two chapters is the lowest. Xu's own medical case histories in these two chapters thus offer illuminating sources of information regarding the social and intellectual contexts in which Xu documented his medical cases, and they help us understand what Xu hoped to achieve.

TABLE 1. Ratios of Xu Shuwei's medical cases to remedies compared with ratios of other peoples' cases to remedies, for every chapter of *The Formulary with Explanatory Historical Contexts.*

Chapter number	Number of remedies	Ratios of Xu's medical cases to remedies (%)	Ratios of other peoples' medical cases to remedies (%)
1	36	17	8
2	45	29	22
3	42	21	12
4	49	12	8
5	39	5	10
6	32	0	13
7	27	11	44
8	25	64	8
9	23	57	0
10	44	19	7

ANECDOTES ABOUT POEMS AND LYRICS

Beginning in the seventh century, medical treatises contained medical case narratives, but Xu Shuwei did not position his *Formulary with Explanatory Historical Contexts* in the genealogy of medical writing. When discussing the inspiration for his formulary, Xu did not mention the fact that some earlier ones collected medical case histories. Yet Xu was far from ignorant of that. Actually, in the main text of *The Formulary with Explanatory Historical Contexts*, he cited case narratives from Shen Kuo's *Good Formulas*, and thus was aware of precedents in formulary writing.[28]

Nonetheless, Xu claimed that he found his inspiration for *The Formulary with Explanatory Historical Contexts* in literary works that gathered narratives of the historical contexts in which a given poem or a lyric was composed or circulated. Xu recalled being inspired as follows:

> Now I am approaching the late stages of my life. I desultorily collected medical formulas I have tested and new ideas I obtained, recording them so as to disseminate them to far distances. I entitle this book *The Widely Benefiting Formulary with Explanatory Historical Contexts*. Meng Qi wrote *Poems with Explanatory Historical Contexts*. Yang Yuansu wrote *Lyrics with Explanatory Historical Contexts*. Both of these works contained "facts at that time" [*dangshi shishi*], so that their readers could see "the twist and unfolding" [*quzhe*] behind their works [i.e., a poem or a lyric]. Given that I devote my heart to saving living beings, and not requesting rewards, how could I not share this formulary with the public?[29]

In mentioning Yang Yuansu's *Lyrics with Explanatory Historical Contexts*, Xu is referring to *A Collection of the Contemporaneously Wise's Lyrics with Explanatory Historical Contexts* (Shixian benshi quziji, hereafter *Lyrics with Explanatory Historical Contexts*) by Yang Hui (1027–1088; his style name was Yuansu). Xu here analogized the meaning of the term *benshi* (explanatory historical contexts or original incidents) in his formulary title with that in Meng Qi's *Poems with Explanatory Historical Contexts* (Benshi shi) and Yang Hui's *Lyrics with Explanatory Historical Contexts*.

Meng Qi completed *Poems with Explanatory Historical Contexts* in 886. It was the first monograph in China that collected anecdotes about a specific Tang poet (including his love affairs) that accounted for the historical contexts in

DEMONSTRATION OF MEDICAL VIRTUOSITY *85*

which a given poem was composed or circulated. Prior to Meng's work, records of the historical contexts appeared occasionally at the beginning of a poem or in a long poem's title; corresponding anecdotes were scattered across entries in novels and notebook-style writings. Meng Qi was the first author to place such contexts and anecdotes together into an independent book.[30]

Scholars have considered Yang Hui's *Lyrics with Explanatory Historical Contexts* to be the monograph that ushered in the "lyric remarks" (*cihua*) genre. Only a dozen entries in this work survive, and most of those record anecdotes about lyric writers and background stories about the composition of a given lyric. Unfortunately, those entries leave us no further information about Yang Hui's rationale for selecting anecdotes to be recorded. Soon after the completion of *Lyrics with Explanatory Historical Contexts*, this work was circulated among literati; for instance, Gao Cheng's *Recording the Origins of Things and Affairs* (Shiwu jiyuan) already cited it in 1080.[31]

The parallel that Xu Shuwei drew between the abovementioned two literary works and his *Formulary with Explanatory Historical Contexts* was by no means incidental. Considering Xu's familiarity with literary genres, evidence of which we see in his advanced-scholars degree, he was in all likelihood aware that *Poems with Explanatory Historical Contexts* was a pioneering work in the "anecdotes about poems" genre and that *Lyrics with Explanatory Historical Contexts* was likewise in the "lyric remarks" genre. The parallel thereby indicated that his formulary was also a pioneering early work, if not the first one, in the "explanatory historical contexts of formularies" genre.[32]

The parallel served not only to mark *The Formulary with Explanatory Historical Contexts* as a pioneering work among books that collected medical cases but also to suggest the function and epistemic focus of case narratives in the formulary. Meng Qi and Xu Shuwei both emphasized the pedagogic function and factuality of the "explanatory historical contexts" they documented. Meng believed that these could help readers to understand the meanings or subtle gist of a poem.[33] In the above quotation, Xu declared that the purpose of documenting the historical contexts was to reveal the "twist and unfolding" behind the creation of poems and lyrics. As for medical formulas recorded in Xu's formulary, the twist and unfolding referred to healing cases narrating the application of a given formula. Xu envisioned that the combination of a given medical formula and a relevant case history would help readers better understand the formula. This pedagogic function of cases that Xu envisioned signals medical authors' heightened awareness of cases as a form of medical

86 CHAPTER THREE

writing, particularly as an epistemic form that was useful for transmitting medical knowledge.

Meng Qi emphasized, when selecting which anecdotes and historical contexts should be recorded, that accounts of strange things that he suspected were not "factual" (*shi*) and vulgar anecdotes should be excluded.[34] Meng was far from the only writer in the ninth century who emphasized not only veracity but also an author's epistemic autonomy in determining it. Both Duan Chengshi in his *Miscellaneous Morsels from Youyang* and Duan Gonglu in his *Northward-Facing Doors* expressed a similar emphasis. Meng Qi's *Poems with Explanatory Historical Contexts* reveals that the emphasis on the reliability of a given text and on an author's epistemic autonomy in notebook-style writings became more pronounced than ever in the ninth century.

In using the phrase "explanatory historical contexts," neither Xu Shuwei nor Meng Qi stressed whether the contexts they recorded were based on their firsthand experience. They used the term in reference to the historical factuality of the contexts—in Xu's words, "the facts at that time" (*dangshi shishi*). One purpose of recording "the facts at that time" was to demonstrate in detail how events took place. In *Poems with Explanatory Historical Contexts* and *Lyrics with Explanatory Historical Contexts*, such events could involve the scenario in which a given poem or lyric was composed. In *The Formulary with Explanatory Historical Contexts*, the events could involve scenarios in which a set of remedies were designed and achieved successful outcomes.

The way in which Xu Shuwei paralleled his formulary with Meng Qi's and Yang Hui's works offers an important clue to Xu's readership targeting. When appealing to the parallel between his composition and Meng's and Yang's, Xu provided no further background information about the two literary works; he merely introduced their book titles and the authors' names. Such a brief introduction implies that Xu assumed that his readers already knew about them and even perhaps recognized them as pioneering pieces conveying anecdotes about poetry and lyrics. Readers with that knowledge would likely have been educated men who were familiar with literary works, such as himself.

In paralleling the three books with explanatory historical contexts, Xu displayed his public persona as an educated figure who was familiar with literary and historical knowledge. This persona implicitly differentiated him from most common physicians. Although Xu had earned his living practicing medicine over several decades, he completed *The Formulary with Explanatory Historical Contexts* only after passing the civil service examination and attaining a position as a civil official. In other words, when Xu completed this formulary, his social status and cultural reputation were both much higher than those of a common physician.

Other hints at the difference between Xu Shuwei and common physicians come from Xu's preface to *The Formulary with Explanatory Historical Contexts*. It began with Xu's praise of medical knowledge: "the 'way' (*dao*) of medicine" is more than "arts" (*yi*) and "techniques" (*ji*), because it could bring the dead back to life. Immediately after offering this praise, Xu then listed the names of eminent physicians from ancient times to the Tang dynasty, such as Sun Simiao, whom Xu regarded as fathoming the way of medicine. Why, Xu wondered, was those physicians' way of medicine much better than medical skills during his time? He answered that it was because in earlier days, physicians practiced medicine for the purpose of saving lives, and Heaven accordingly gifted the way of medicine to them; in contrast, contemporaneous physicians thought only of profits, and Heaven consequently refused to bestow the way of medicine upon them. Xu then argued that the lack of competent physicians in his home county caused his parents' deaths when he was a child. "Being anguished by the thought that there was not a single good physician in our village [who could help my parents]," Xu began to learn medicine and "swore wholeheartedly to devote my life to saving all living beings."[35] By narrating his question, answer, and vow in this sequence, Xu implied that his way of medicine was better than that of contemporaneous physicians because he aimed to save lives, while the others aimed to earn money. At the end of the preface, Xu stated again that he saved lives without seeking rewards. This statement reminded his readers of the contradiction between what he regarded as eminent and common physicians that he had mentioned earlier.

Xu's inclusion of the phrase "explanatory historical contexts" (*benshi*) in his formulary title merits special attention. This phrasing marks the first time that language referring to medical case narratives, which usually appeared in prefaces and postscripts, was included in a book title. The parallel that Xu Shuwei drew between *The Formulary with Explanatory Historical Contexts* and the other two literary works had multiple implications. For one thing, the title indicated that his treatise on the collection of medical case histories was a pioneering work, thus attracting educated men as his target audience and fashioning Xu as a learned and benevolent medical expert.

Although Xu's use of the term "explanatory historical contexts" bore similarities to Meng Qi's use of the phrase, one of Xu's remarks in his preface helps us differentiate his formulary from Meng's works, that is, the inclusion of "new ideas" (*xinyi*) that Xu acquired over his long career in healing. Meng stressed in his preface his efforts to verify the historical contexts he recorded; he gave no word regarding any his creative labors.[36] In contrast, Xu pointed out that his formulary not only collected relevant historical contexts but also presented his new ideas about healing. In this regard, Xu Shuwei demonstrated the more prominent presence of his discoveries and intellectual voice in his formulary compared with Meng's.

MEDICAL CASES AND PHYSICIANS' FAME

When Xu Shuwei was writing his medical treatises, the scope and purposes of collecting medical case histories underwent a significant change. The appearance of a particular formulary in the early twelfth century marked this new development. The formulary, *Straightforward Rhymes of Medicines for and Syndromes of Children* (Xiaoer yaozheng zhijue, or *Authentic Rhymes of Medicines for and Syndromes of Children*, Xiaoer yaozheng zhenjue, hereafter *Straightforward Rhymes*), devoted an entire chapter (*juan*) to presenting a single physician's case histories. In comparison, from the seventh century onward, a growing number of authors published formularies that contained medical case narratives, but they scattered case records throughout a given book. Those formularies included *Essential Formulas, Mr. Cui's Collections of Essential Formulas,* and *Passing on Trustworthy Formulas,* as discussed in chapter 1.

The sole physician who was subject to depiction in *Straightforward Rhymes'* case histories was Qian Yi (ca. 1032–1113), a famous pediatrician. Qian won great fame and served as a medical official at the court after curing Emperor Shenzong's niece during the Yuanfeng reign (1078–1085). Nonetheless, the author of *Straightforward Rhymes* was not Qian but one of his patients, Yan Jizhong.

Yan's preface to *Straightforward Rhymes* reveals alternative, even contradictory, views on the usefulness of publishing medical case histories that were being expressed by the time of fall of the Northern Song empire. According to the preface, Qian Yi had cured Yan when he was five or six years old and was about to die from multiple diseases. Qian was young at that time and "not willing to transmit his writings casually."[37] Even after Qian became a renowned court medical official—the peak of a physician's career in the Song era—he still did not complete and publish a medical treatise. Qian's doubt about the helpfulness of transmitting medical knowledge via a documentary format was reminiscent of Shen Kuo's belief that one could not fathom medicine only by reading books (a belief analyzed in chapter 1). Regardless of Qian's doubt, Yan was determined to collect and publish Qian's notes on pediatric knowledge. He spent decades collecting the relevant materials, such as Qian's medical essays and formulas, from his own relatives and acquaintances. Yan also found "other versions" (*bieben*) of Qian's writings that were circulating in Kaifeng. He then compared them and edited all of the materials he had collected so painstakingly, reorganizing them into *Straightforward Rhymes*.

Yan Jizhong organized Qian Yi's materials in the pattern of a discussion-case-prescription trilogy. He structured *Straightforward Rhymes* into three chapters. The first includes some 47 medical "discussions" (*lun*) about pediatrics. The second lists twenty-three case-based accounts, identifying them as "Records of Twenty-Three Disorders Qian Yi Once Treated." The third chapter lists some 114 medical formulas. As modern scholarship has observed, the discussion-case-prescription trilogy format indicates that Qian's case histories were more likely read as an explanatory chapter supporting the preceding chapter of medical discussions and the following chapter of formulas.[38]

The general structure and form that some of the episodes among the twenty-three case records take are similar to the that of Xu Shuwei's cases. Both follow a basic pattern in which a patient's personal information is related before describing the disorders in question and relevant medical histories, eventually accounting for their diagnosis and prescription before noting the outcome for the patient. This structure is commonplace in case histories in earlier texts, such as Chunyu Yi's examination records from the second century BCE and Sun Simiao's *Essential Formulas* in the early seventh century CE. Like Xu in his case histories, Qian Yi in his acknowledges fierce competition for patient patronage. Qian often had to debate rival healers and persuade opinionated members of patients' households to earn their patronage. The medical debates and Qian's successful cures portrayed in the twenty-three cases validated Yan's assessment of Qian's extraordinary healing skills.

The appearance of *Straightforward Rhymes* suggests that publishing formularies in the discussion-case-prescription trilogy format became a means of demonstrating a physician's medical virtuosity and bolstering his fame as a successful practitioner. Such a trilogy is evident in Xu Shuwei's own medical case narratives as well, especially those that involve cold damage disorders. The special attention that Xu paid to gathering his cases of cold damage disorders grew out of the development of this medical subfield in his time.

CANONIZATION AND POPULARIZATION

Cold damage medicine rose in salience in the Song era, as indicated by the soaring number of medical treatises that were specific to this medical subfield. Approximately ten of this sort had been published before the Song dynasty, a period spanning seven hundred years, running from the third to the tenth centuries, whereas there were sixty-five in the Song era.[39] Modern scholars have proposed various explanations for the rise of cold damage medicine during this period, such as frequent outbreaks of epidemics in China.[40] Another explanation cites the unusually cold climate experienced between 985 and 1192.[41] One significant contributing factor that scholars have agreed upon is the canonization and popularization during the Song dynasty of a third-century formulary, *Treatise on Cold Damage*. Beyond this consensus, however, the specific process involved in and the timeline of the canonization and popularization of this formulary are unclear. Issues under debate, for instance, include how the treatise became widely known among medical authors across China, and when medical authors began to acclaim it as a canon of cold damage medicine. Resolving these issues would require comprehensive research into both received and excavated sources in middle-period China, a project deserving of an entire monograph on its own. Here, our focus is on the trajectory over which the treatise was considered a cold damage canon and on the process in which this concept prevailed in the Song era.

The received story about the birth of *Treatise on Cold Damage* began with its author Zhang Ji's (150?–219?) great loss of his "kinsmen" (*zongzu*), who originally numbered some two hundred people. During the Jian'an reign (196–220), two-thirds of his kinsmen died within the span of a single decade. Of those, seven of ten died of cold damage.[42] This great loss drove Zhang to study medicine diligently and search widely to collect remedies, completing *Treatise on Cold Damage and Miscellaneous Disorders* (Shanghan zabing lun, hereafter *Cold Damage and Miscellaneous Disorders*) sometime between 202 and 217. This story about epidemics originates from a preface to it, which is attributed to Zhang Ji. Medical historians have hotly debated whether Zhang was the author of the preface; they have also disputed its accuracy.[43] As shown in a recent discussion, this story about epidemics appeared in the Song era, eight hundred years after

Zhang's death. Another issue that has been subject to debate among medical historians is whether Zhang served as the governor of Changsha (in Hunan).[44] No evidence in the Han dynasty can be found to prove this; however, the Song literati believed that Zhang was the governor.

As signaled in the title, *Cold Damage and Miscellaneous Diseases* classified disorders into two large categories: one covered cold damage disorders and the other covered all the other types of disorders that Zhang collectively called "miscellaneous disorders." Along the lines of transmission over the centuries, the two disorder-category parts of *Cold Damage and Miscellaneous Disorders* became separated from each other, circulating as independent treatises. The one on cold damage disorders is what the Song people called *Treatise on Cold Damage.*

According to the received view, *Treatise on Cold Damage* was not circulated widely from the third to the eleventh centuries.[45] Scholars have reported that, even in the early seventh century, it circulated among only a small group of physicians in Jiangnan, the area south of the Yangzi River; it was not until the Directorate of Education printed this text in 1065 and 1088 that it became widely available and accessible to physicians and literati. Based on this view, the medical historian Asaf Goldschmidt's research took this understanding a step further and proposed a key change in Song medicine. To simplify Goldschmidt's argument greatly, the newly available *Treatise on Cold Damage* stimulated physicians in the Song era to integrate theories in this ancient treatise with contemporary healing practices; their pursuit of this integration fostered the emergence of a great number of treatises specific to cold damage medicine. The integration characterizes the Song era as one of the three turning points in the development of Chinese medicine.[46] Goldschmidt's argument has been influential and over the past decade has provoked an intense discussion on the evolution of cold damage medicine in middle-period China.

Recent studies have seriously challenged the foregoing received view. They show that, before 1065, when the directorate printed the entire contents of *Treatise on Cold Damage,* parts of this book were already circulating widely; medical treatises completed between the third and seventh centuries had drawn formulas from it.[47] For instance, Sun Simiao had transcribed parts of it in his *Supplement to Formulas Worth a Thousand in Gold.*[48] Treatises whose titles contained the term "cold damage" and were attributed to Zhang Ji appeared continuously in other medical texts and bibliographies in the Six Dynasties and Tang eras, such as *Discerning Cold Damage* (Bian shanghan). Those cold damage treatises that were attributed to Zhang presumably drew their sources from part of the cold damage treatments recorded in *Treatise on Cold Damage* and *Cold Damage and Miscellaneous Diseases*.[49] In other words, the circulation of the former from the third to the eleventh centuries, even though it was not in a complete book version, was wider than previous scholarship has thought. This meant that the contents of *Treatise on Cold Damage* for physicians in the Song era may not have been as new as the received view suggested.

In addition to challenging the received view, which tended to emphasize the quick and direct influence of the directorate-printed *Treatise on Cold Damage* as boosting cold damage medicine in the Song era, recent studies have also presented a less linear trajectory of its canonization and popularization in this period. They have pointed out the more limited circulation of the directorate-printed version and the popularity of an easy-to-understand guidebook on *Treatise on Cold Damage*. The directorate printed the treatise in 1065 and 1088, assigning it as a textbook in government medical education and examinations by 1083.[50] Beyond that government system, physicians may have encountered difficulties in accessing the directorate-printed version.

Unlike what the rapid spread of *Treatise on Cold Damage* in government medical education implies, however, not every early Northern Song medical treatise that was completed in private hands and specific to cold damage cited it. One example is *Master Tongzhen's Summary of Cold Damage* (Tongzhen zi shanghan kuoyao), which was attributed to Liu Yuanbin (fl. 1076–1090), the assistant magistrate of Shaoyang County in Shao Prefecture (in Hunan). The first half of the extant version of *Master Tongzhen's Summary of Cold Damage* drew primarily from the Song court–compiled *The Imperial Grace Formulary* instead of *Treatise on Cold Damage*.[51] Beginning in 1088, the second time the directorate printed *Treatise on Cold Damage*, and running to the end of the Southern Song dynasty, little evidence suggests that this treatise was reprinted as an independent book.

In comparison with the dissemination of *Treatise on Cold Damage*, an easy-to-understand guide to it, *One Hundred Questions on Cold Damage* (1107, hereafter *One Hundred Questions*), circulated more widely. As shown in recent studies, it was instrumental in achieving the canonization and popularization of *Treatise on Cold Damage* in the Song period. Its author, Zhu Gong, used the question-and-answer format to elaborate the content of the treatise, posing 101 questions about applying it to healing practices. Zhu then appended answers after each question. For instance, the questions involved factors such as when specific symptoms (such as feeling cold limbs) manifested and a specific pulse pattern was diagnosed or what drug therapies could be applied. In answering those questions, Zhu recommended pertinent drug therapies and explained the rationale for each prescription.

Zhu took twenty years to complete *One Hundred Questions*. He claimed in 1107 that he had written a book that explained the content of *Treatise on Cold Damage* so that "scholar-officials would easily understand it and subsequently enjoy reading it."[52] In the early twelfth century, when Zhu was retired, he moved to West Lake (in Zhejiang) and continued writing the book. He completed his efforts in 1107.[53] Four years later, Zhu Gong assigned his son to submit *One Hundred Questions* to the court and requested that the court print it.[54] In 1114, when Emperor Huizong's government was promoting the status of medicine, it appointed Zhu Gong as "erudite master" of the medical academy.

Parts of *One Hundred Questions* were circulating before Zhu Gong's son submitted the entire book to the court in 1111. Before then, Zhang Chan, who presumably was a physician, claimed that he had read a treatise entitled *Mr. Seeking Nothing's One Hundred Questions on Cold Damage* (Wuqiuzi shanghan baiwen) in what is now the southeast region of Jiangsu.[55] At that point, Zhang had no idea who the author—Mr. Seeking Nothing (or Mr. Not Seeking Fame and Wealth, *Wuqiuzi*)—was. When he met Zhu Gong around West Lake in Hangzhou, he found out that Zhu was Mr. Seeking Nothing and that what he read was merely 60 percent of the contents of Zhu's original *One Hundred Questions*. Zhang received the entire version from Zhu and edited it. The outcome of Zhang's editing was a treatise of twenty chapters and some ninety-one thousand words. Zhang named the treatise *The Book for Saving Lives from Nanyang* (Nanyang huoren shu, hereafter *Saving Lives*). Nanyang, in this title, as Zhang Chan explained, referred to Zhang Ji and his oeuvre, because Nanyang was Zhang Ji's home county.

Saving Lives was printed many times across Song China after the early twelfth century. In 1116, Zhu Gong retired and returned to Hangzhou. On his way there, he heard that *Saving Lives* had been printed in the capital Kaifeng, Chengdu, Hunan, Fujian, and Liangzhe (in Jiangsu); one of the publishers of the printed versions in Kaifeng might have been the Directorate of Education.[56] It was a pity, his informants complained to Zhu, that those printed versions were not properly edited and were full of mistakes. After returning to Hangzhou, Zhu made some one hundred revisions to *Saving Lives* and asked a commercial publisher in Hangzhou to print this version in 1118.[57] In 1176, "the previous versions" (*jiuben*, perhaps not the version revised by Zhu Gong) of *Saving Lives* were printed "among laymen" (*minjian*) in Jian Prefecture (in Fujian) and Rao Prefecture (in Jiangxi); the prefectural office (*gongshiku*) in Chi Prefecture (in Anhui) printed Zhu's revised version.[58]

The ample number of printed editions and the wide geographical scope of the printings of *Saving Lives* attest to its popularity in Song China. This meant that many more readers learned about *Treatise on Cold Damage* by reading Zhu Gong's easy-to-understand guidebook. In addition to popularizing the treatise, *Saving Lives* was the first extant source that explicitly added *Treatise on Cold Damage* to the "canon" (*jing*) of cold damage medicine.[59] Medical authors had praised it before Zhu did. The first surviving reference to Zhang Ji as a sage appeared in the preface to the directorate-printed version, written by civil officials who were in charge of this editing project.[60] Nevertheless, Zhu was one of the earliest authors to extol it as a contribution to the medical canon. Following publication of *Saving Lives*, a growing number of medical authors began advocating for including *Treatise on Cold Damage* in the canon of cold damage medicine.

Xu Shuwei's treatises likewise contributed to the trend toward canonizing and popularizing *Treatise on Cold Damage*. Goldschmidt proposed that three cold damage treatises attributed to Xu were probably intended to be read together as a trilogy so as to make *Treatise on Cold Damage* easier for nonexperts to understand. The first part, *One Hundred Mnemonic Verses on Cold Damage Manifestations*, consists of one hundred rhymes, each of which summarizes parts of *Treatise on Cold Damage*. The second, *Subtleties of Cold Damage Revealed*, consists of twenty-two "discussions" (*lun*). In each of the discussions, Xu talks about one topic concerning the diagnosis and treatment of a cold damage disorder. The third part, *Ninety Discussions*, consists of Xu's ninety medical cases of these disorders. Goldschmidt formulated the trilogy in such a way that each of the three books, in its specific written form (i.e., rhymes, discussions, and cases) popularized *Treatise on Cold Damage* in a distinct way: *One Hundred Mnemonic Verses* transformed its contents into easy-to-remember rhymes, *Subtleties of Cold Damage Revealed* discussed the important but difficult-to-understand medical issues it mentioned, and by documenting Xu's healing practice, *Ninety Discussions* merged the ancient medical theories mentioned in the treatise with Xu's clinical practice, demonstrating how to apply the third-century classic to twelfth-century healing practices.[61] Taken together, the three books made *Treatise on Cold Damage* more comprehensible to a wider audience.

Although the identification, in existing scholarship, of Xu Shuwei as the author of *Ninety Discussions* appears to be erroneous, the trilogy that Goldschmidt proposed has inspired the present study to view Xu's medical cases of cold damage disorders in *The Formulary with Explanatory Historical Contexts* as contributing to his advocacy of *Treatise on Cold Damage* as a cold damage classic and as a way of popularizing the book. Findings in recent studies also modify the trilogy, showing that, in addition to *Treatise on Cold Damage*, another cold damage treatise that Xu's books promoted was *Saving Lives*. For instance, although Xu claimed that everything in his *One Hundred Mnemonic Verses* "originated from Zhang Zhongjing," two-thirds of its rhymes actually summarized Zhu Gong's words in *Saving Lives*.[62]

The abovementioned studies on the development of cold damage medicine in the Song era focused on progress toward canonization and popularization of cold damage medical treatises and the integration of medical theories and practice. Disputes arose however, over the course of this canonization, popularization, and integration.

MEDICAL DEBATES

Xu Shuwei wrote and published cases involving cold damage in response to disputes over the diagnosis of and prescriptions for these disorders that arose in the course of the canonization and popularization of *Treatise on Cold Damage*. These disputes manifested in three ways: debates involving clinical encounters with assembled rival healers or members of patients' households; Xu's ongoing discussion with a figure whom he did not identify, where it is often difficult to discern whether the discussion took place in a clinical setting; and an intertextual debate between Xu and other contemporaneous authors, which was a relatively new phenomenon in the Song era. The three types of disputes mark *The Formulary with Explanatory Historical Contexts* as a pioneering treatise in China whose author deliberately marshaled his case histories to support his opinions in medical debates, either in clinical practice or in intertextual space.

The debates involved in Xu's clinical encounters often began with questions raised by assembled physicians and a patient's family regarding the justification for a diagnosis and prescription. These ranged from wanting to know the names of disorders to wondering about remedies Xu recommended to puzzlement over seemingly worsening manifestations in a patient who had consumed one

96 CHAPTER THREE

of Xu's remedies. One example of such a debate is exhibited in the case narrative with which this chapter opens. In it, the assembled physicians doubted why Xu chose to use the Major Bupleurum Decoction instead of a honey enema.

If challenges to a prescription came from members of a patient's household, Xu sometimes did not answer them orally in a clinical setting. Instead, he included the complaints and his justifications in a written case narrative in *The Formulary with Explanatory Historical Contexts*. Here is a typical example: When examining a patient named Mr. Qiu from Xu's hometown, Xu said: "Although this is a manifestation type of Ephedra [Decoction], the pulse at the 'foot position' (*chi*) is tardy and weak. *Treatise on Cold Damage* says: 'If the pulse at the foot position is tardy, it is because the "nutrient qi" (*rongqi*) is insufficient and the "blood" (*xue*) and the qi are very scant. One cannot sweat the patient at this moment.'"[63] Accordingly, Xu did not sweat Mr. Qiu. Xu prepared a "Construct the Middle Decoction" (Jianzhong Tang), adding Chinese angelica and astragalus (*huangqi*), and ordered Mr. Qiu to drink it. Even though Xu explained the rationale for his prescription, the next day, members of Mr. Qiu's household became impatient and kept urging Xu to administer a diaphoretic drug. Their language even approached rudeness. "I put up with this [abuse]," Xu recalled in his response in the case narrative. Not ingratiating himself with those rude family members, Xu stick to his original prescription plan. After some five days, Mr. Qiu was cured.

Following this successful outcome, Xu in the case narrative cautioned physicians against applying treatments in the wrong sequence. He warned, "I often saw that patients' household members were impatient. The patient was sick no more than three or four days, and they urged physicians, day and night, to apply sweating treatment." Once physicians comply with household members' ignorant opinions, treatments often fail. "Therefore," Xu noted, "I document this as a special word of caution for physicians."[64] Although he claimed that the caution was written for physicians, it could also have been intended simultaneously to educate his readers to heed the proper timing for sweating a patient who suffered similar symptoms.

When replying to rival healers' questions and justifying his own diagnoses and prescriptions, Xu frequently interpreted medical classics. He also used this method to justify his treatments in other types of dispute. For instance, in one case record, a person suffered from dysentery, his body felt hot, his mind was clouded, he raved, and he could not fall asleep. Xu palpated the patient's pulse and said, "This was the manifestation type of Minor Order-the-Qi Decoction" (Xiao Chengqi Tang)." Observers were astounded by this diagnosis, asking, "Can prescribing Minor Order-the-Qi Decoction for dysentery be one of *Treatise on Cold Damage*'s methods?" Xu answered: "This is the method in *Treatise on Cold Damage*. It says, 'Patients have dysentery, raved, and have dried excrement. This belongs to the manifestation type of Minor Order-the-Qi Decoction.' I once read *Basic Questions*. It says, 'When the disorder is slight, go against it; when it is strong, conform to it. Going against the pathogen means treating it directly; following it means treating it contrarily.'"[65] Here Xu cited *Treatise on Cold Damage* and *Basic Questions* to legitimize his prescription.

Next to *Treatise on Cold Damage*, *Basic Questions* is the second most frequently cited medical classic that Xu used to support his positions in medical debates. *Basic Questions* and *Divine Pivot* together constitute *The Yellow Emperor's Inner Canon* (Huangdi neijing, hereafter *The Inner Canon*), which has long been considered the most crucial work in classical medicine in imperial China and, even today, occupies the role of a textbook in curricula on traditional Chinese medicine. The earliest compilation presumably dated from the Han dynasty, though it is not the oldest medical text in China; archaeological excavations since the 1980s have discovered older materials. *The Inner Canon* is, however, the oldest extant work of literature recognized as a source of canonical medical doctrine in China.[66]

In Xu Shuwei's medical cases, physicians of his day were less familiar with *Treatise on Cold Damage* and other medical classics than Xu was; Xu often won debates by drawing references from them. It should not be surprising, though, that Xu exaggerated his rival healers' ignorance of medical classics to makes his erudition conspicuous. But did he really persuade rival healers and patients' household members in clinical practice by appealing to medical classics? Or did he construct this plot to promote his own erudition? To what degree and on what grounds can we consider Xu's medical cases as narrated as accurate depictions of what actually happened in clinical practice? Given the dearth of other evidence, it is difficult to give these questions concrete answers.[67] What we know for certain is that, in his medical cases, Xu used his success in practice and textual learning as the underpinning of his expertise in medicine.

After describing debates and successful outcomes in clinical practice, Xu sometimes notes that "one may ask" (*huowen*) or "one may say" (*huoyue*) regarding a given question, followed by a reply to the question. Considering that passages in this dialogic form often appear following accounts of outcomes and in the absence of questioners' names or personal information, it seems that Xu had no intention of identifying the participants in dialogues that took place in clinical settings. Instead, they were designed to function more like conversations between Xu and his readers, thus they may be differentiated from medical debates occurring in clinical settings and be counted as the second type of dispute included in Xu's medical cases. Some discussions of this type are similar to those raised by assembled physicians, which mainly concerned the rationale for a given diagnosis and prescription. Others express confusion of the sort that readers might experience when reading *Treatise on Cold Damage*, such as that involving paradoxical prescriptions and the meanings of medical terminology. One typical example stems from the case narrative involving the Major Bupleurum Decoction, in which Xu noted questions from unidentified figures: "In discussing Yang Brightness disorder, Zhongjing says, 'In the case of those with profuse sweating, urgently drain the patient's bodily fluid downward.' Many people often say that when the patient is spontaneously sweating and one further drains the patient's bodily fluid downward, how could the result not be depletion in both the interior and exterior aspects of the body?"[68] To answer this question, Xu elaborated on his interpretation of Zhang Ji's words. The successful outcome that preceded this question and answer enhanced the credibility of Xu's interpretation.

Transmitting knowledge through the question-and-answer form was a long-standing practice in medical literature in China, whereas in the twelfth-century, sources of authority in this form differed markedly from those cited in ancient times. The dialogue form can be traced back to *Basic Questions*; as shown in its title, this form constitutes the primary means of passing down knowledge. In this medical classic, divine figures, such the Yellow Emperor, asked questions about medical knowledge, and another legendary figure answered at length. The authority of those answers derived not from their authorship, which was often obscured in ancient medical treatises, but from the associated legendary figures. In contrast, in twelfth-century medical treatises, the authors rarely identified questioners' names or personal information in a dialogue, and sources of the authority supporting the answers were closely associated with the authorship of a treatise. For instance, Zhu Gong, the author of *Saving Lives*, gained much of that authority from his court appointment as the "erudite master" of the medical academy; Xu Shuwei in *The Formulary with Explanatory Historical Contexts* based its authority largely on his successful practice and medical erudition.

Xu, when elaborating his interpretation of *Treatise on Cold Damage* to un-identified questioners, sometimes commented on his contemporaneous cold damage treatises. Intertextual dialogues with contemporaneous medical authors such as this constitute a third type of medical dispute in Xu's cases. These dialogues seldom appeared in earlier medical literature but proliferated in the Song era. One case in point is Zhang Chan's 1111 preface to *Saving Lives*. When praising the book, Zhang hinted that he had also read five other Northern Song authors' cold damage texts. The dates of the five attest to the short period of time between the publication of a Song cold damage treatise and its entry in intertextual dialogues between contemporaneous writers; they are *Classified and Collected Cold Damage Disorders* (Shanghan zuanlei) by Gao Roune (977–1055), *Alternative Orders of Cold Damage Disorders* (Bieci shanghan) by Shen Kuo, *Classified Examples of Cold Damage Disorders* (Shanghan leili) by Hu Mian (fl. ca. 11th century), *Rhymed Instructions on the Pulse Patterns of Cold Damage Disorders* (Shanghan maijue) by Sun Zhao (fl. 11th century), and *Discussions on Cold Damage and General Disorders* (Shanghan zongbing lun) by Pang Anshi (1042–1099).[69] Those five treatises, Zhang Chan commented, introduced innovations yet were less organized than *Saving Lives*.

The Formulary with Explanatory Historical Contexts abounds with intertextual dialogues with contemporaneous authors, such as Wang Shi (fl. ca. 11th century), Sun Zhao, Pang Anshi, and, of course, Zhu Gong. In the dialogues, Xu Shuwei sometimes concurred with their opinions but sometimes expressed his disagreement with them very directly. In one case, for example, someone asked Xu about the pathological course of cold damage disorders in the body. Xu replied, in a matter-of-fact tone, that neither *Treatise on Cold Damage* nor previous or present texts discuss the pathological course; only Pang Anshi proposed a course and a rationale. After reiterating the course and rationale, Xu explicitly refuted it by saying, "I consider it is wrong" and "It is so contrived." Xu then cited a sentence from *Basic Questions* to support his refutation.[70]

Pang Anshi was a physician who was active in eleventh-century Hubei and was famous for cold damage medicine. Xu's refutation of Pang's views is noteworthy, because it shows that disputes over cold damage medicine arose not only between physicians and laymen or between eminent healers and incompetent ones but also between doctors who specialized in this medical subfield. No one's medical authority was self-evidently preeminent.

Another example of Xu's case records involving intertextual dialogues concerns the meaning of cold damage medical terminology. This case record illustrates the difficulty of learning this medicine by reading books without intermediaries. In it, Xu examined a patient who suffered from a cold damage disorder but who did not sweat and had an aversion to wind, and whose neck was bent but rigid. Xu said, "This condition is called 'neck rigidity and *jiji*.' The manifestation type of the Kudzu Decoction (Gegen Tang)." Immediately after recording this diagnosis, Xu writes: "One may ask 'What is meant by *jiji*?' I said: '*Jiji* refers to a condition similar to one when a patient suffers a foot disorder and their feet [or legs] are bent but rigid. Xie Fugu, when he referred to this term, said that it means a condition in which the patient is so sick and feeble that he must lean on a desk to rise. It is wrong.'"[71]

Xie Fugu was a Song-dynasty medical author and served as the academician of the Hanlin Academy. Xu did not explain why he objected to Xie's understanding of the term *jiji*; perhaps he thought the mistake was too obvious. But at the end of the entry, Xu notes that "there are many points in *Treatise on Cold Damage* that were difficult to comprehend" and lists five other phrases as examples.

Notably, in this intertextual dialogue, Xu did not bestow greater intellectual authority on the court-commissioned version of *Treatise on Cold Damage*, which the Bureau for Editing Medical Texts edited and the Directorate of Education printed. Rather, Xu criticized its comments on the treatise. His criticism appears in his reply to an unidentified questioner's doubt about his prescription: "The patient has already vomited and was then treated by draining his bodily fluid downward; this is a case of internal depletion. How can you apply White Tiger Decoction [Baihu Tang]?" In response, Xu cited two sentences in *Treatise on Cold Damage* and elaborated their meaning. At the end of his elaboration, Xu criticized the bureau's comment on the two sentences: "Our dynasty's Lin Yi, in his critical edition of *Treatise on Cold Damage*, wrote: 'Zhang Zhongjing in detailing this method wrote the words "exterior" and "interior" incorrectly.' I said it was not the case."[72] Lin Yi was one of the three civil officials who were in charge of the bureau's editing project for *Treatise on Cold Damage*.

Xu went on to explain why Lin was wrong and concluded his criticism of the bureau's comments on the treatise as follows: "Lin Yi examined only the so-called difference between the interior and exterior aspects of the body and then said there was an error. This was Lin's error due to not thinking it through."[73]

Xu's criticism here is significant. It shows that the appearance of the court-commissioned version of *Treatise on Cold Damage* by no means quelled Song authors' frequent and wide-ranging debates over the diagnosis and prescription of cold damage disorders and over the correct understanding of it. The court-commissioned version, some Song authors believed, was nothing but another voice in those battles.

Although the annotations in the court-commissioned version of *Treatise on Cold Damage* did not prove to be sufficiently authoritative to quell the heated debates, that version may help in standardizing the treatise's contents. Recent scholarship has observed that, before the directorate printed the version of *Essential Formulas* that the Bureau for Editing Medical Texts had edited, medical treatises had asserted various opinions about when menarche would begin, ranging from fourteen to sixteen years of age. After the court-commissioned version of *Essential Formulas* was issued—which stated that menarche began when a female reached fourteen—other versions of *Essential Formulas* followed suit.[74] The court-commissioned version of *Treatise on Cold Damage* could function similarly in the effort to standardize the contents of this canonical medical work.

AS AN EARLY PIONEERING WORK that groups medical case histories as supportive evidence in medical debates, *The Formulary with Explanatory Historical Contexts* had multiple inspirations. The core inspiration that its author, Xu Shuwei, claimed was not medical writing but literary works: *Poems with Explanatory Historical Contexts* and *Lyrics with Explanatory Historical Contexts*. The analogy drawn in Xu's preface between those and his formulary had several implications. It illustrated his acquaintance with Tang and Song literary genres, suggesting that his target audience comprised educated men who were familiar with such writings. The analogy meanwhile connoted that *The Formulary with Explanatory Historical Contexts* was a pioneering work in which medical cases constituted a large proportion of the text. By including the phrase "explanatory historical context" (*benshi*) in the title of the formulary, Xu displayed a heightened awareness that his medical predecessors lacked the use of cases as an epistemic form for conveying new knowledge.

In addition to *Poems with Explanatory Historical Contexts* and *Lyrics with Explanatory Historical Contexts*, two changes in social and intellectual contexts encouraged Xu to marshal medical case histories in his formulary. One was the rising visibility of case narratives in medical literature in the early twelfth century, when formulary authors for the first time devoted independent sections to recording a physician's case histories. One formulary, *Straightforward*

Rhymes, provided a precedent for using the discussion-case-prescription trilogy format to build up a physician's fame.

The other change was the diverse and abundant disputes about the understanding of *Treatise on Cold Damage* and cold damage medicine. These arose over the course of the canonization and popularization of the treatise in the eleventh and twelfth centuries, which made the need to understand its medical terminology and theories all the more acute, as compared with its reception in the preceding centuries. Meanwhile, amplified by woodblock printing, the wider dissemination of *Treatise on Cold Damage* and other Song-era cold damage texts meant that contrasting understandings of the treatise and cold damage medicine were more visible to readers in this period than they had been before. The ever more acute need to understand the treatise, along with the growing visibility of contrasting understandings, together encouraged closer intertextual dialogues, sometimes even debates, between medical authors than ever before. To convince readers and prospective dialogue participants of the correctness of their understandings, the Song authors creatively applied a range of persuasion strategies. The key strategy, for example, that Zhu Gong adopted was to seek imperial endorsement of his *Saving Lives*. As for Xu Shuwei, he appealed to the empirical strategy, publishing his collections of case histories. Xu recorded his successful cures and populated his cases with learned remarks. *The Formulary with Explanatory Historical Contexts* was therefore written for publication and to bolster his fame both as a successful practitioner and as an erudite scholar.

The explanatory function of Xu Shuwei's medical cases involving cold damage disorders additionally gives us a glimpse into the use of the medical case narrative in a specific medical subfield during the Song period. In this subfield, where consensus over its canonical sets, such as treatises on cold damage medicine, was being reached, the case narrative in general served to illustrate canonical textual knowledge. In stark contrast, in other medical subfields that lacked such texts, medical case histories played more important roles in bolstering the reliability and credibility of a given treatise and new healing knowledge, a phenomenon examined in the next chapter.

FOUR The Search for Therapies in the Far South

In this year [1131], I suffered seriously from miasma disorders. I applied drugs, which warmed the interior of the body, solidified the lower body parts, caused yin and yang to ascend or descend in the body, and rectified the qi of the body. I used moxibustion on three points on the body, which were *zhongwan, qihai,* and *sanli.*
—Li Qiu, "Li daizhi *Zhangnüe lun,*" in *Lingnan weisheng fang, shang,* 3

THE ABOVE ACCOUNT appears in *Treatise on Zhang [Miasma] and Intermittent Fever* (Zhangnüe lun, hereafter *Treatise on Zhang*), a formulary that was devoted to the treatment of endemic disorders in Lingnan, in far southern China.[1] It was written by a civil official, Li Qiu (?–1151), sometime between 1131 and 1139. In middle-period medical treatises, *zhang* referred either to a pervasive and harmful miasmatic atmosphere or to a category of diseases encompassing a range of symptoms; the above quotation refers to the latter. In *Treatise on Zhang,* Li articulates his opinions on the etiology of and remedies for *zhang* ("miasma") disorders. To support those opinions, he provides detailed accounts of his experience with local healing practices in Lingnan. Those accounts display Li's efforts there to develop remedies that could treat fatal and *zhang* disorders. Li was far from the only official who was posted to Lingnan and sought effective treatments, as his formulary soon stimulated officials' production of new medical texts on southern disorders that continued over the following decades. One such is Wang Fei's *Formulary for Instructing the Lost and on Zhang [Miasma] and Intermittent Fever* (Zhimi fang zhangnüe lun, hereafter *Instructing the Lost*). Like Li Qiu, Wang used his experience in Lingnan to support what he wrote about the etiology of and treatments for *zhang* disorders.

Two crucial factors contributed to Song officials' application of the empirical strategy in their formularies on far-southern disorders. One is what they regarded as a lack of reliable medical texts and remedies for treating disorders occurring in Lingnan. The other is the popular practice in middle-period China whereby officials who had lived in Lingnan recorded their experiences in the region, especially those that reflected local customs and the warm, humid environment.

ZHANG AS MIASMA AND SOUTHERN DISORDERS

Zhang was one of the most frequently discussed families of far-southern disorders in imperial China, from the earliest written records that mention it in the fifth century to its treatment in the Song era.[2] Its Chinese character, understood as denoting epidemics occurring in the south, can be traced to the fifth century. Before then, this character appeared neither in excavated early manuscripts nor in *The Inner Canon*, which is the oldest of any medical texts considered canonical and contains materials dating to the Han era.[3] The character for *zhang* appears, for example, in the biography of Ma Yuan (d. 49 CE), which Fan Ye wrote as part of a standard history, *History of the Later Han* (Hou Han shu), and presented it to the court in 445 CE. According to the biography, Emperor Guangwu (5 BCE–57 CE, r. 25–55 CE) commissioned Ma in 42 CE to suppress a rebellion on the far-southern border, in Jiaozhi (now the northern area of Vietnam). When he was there, Ma often consumed coix seeds (*yiyishi*) to overcome the "miasmatic atmosphere" (*zhangqi*).[4] In the autumn of 44 CE, after Ma's armies quashed the rebellion, approximately 40–50 percent of the soldiers involved died in *zhang* epidemics (*zhangyi*).[5] The biography used the character for *zhang* to refer to the miasmatic atmosphere and fatal epidemics but introduced no explanations of what might have triggered them.

A report by Yang Zhong to Emperor Zhang (57–88 CE, r. 75–88) in 76 CE (another record in *History of the Later Han*) used the term *zhang* to denote obstacles, when referring to a debilitating issue arising from the southern environment. In the report, Yang said: "The south is 'summer hot' (*shu*) and damp; 'obstacles' (*zhang*) and 'the toxic' (*du*) give rise to each other."[6] Yang used this explanation to persuade Emperor Zhang not to exile political criminals to the remote southern areas of China. By extension, in his report, the character for *zhang* was used in reference to disorders that were specific to the south to discourage migration. Yang ascribed the southern-specific disorders to the "summer heat" (*shu*) and dampness in that region.[7]

After the Eastern Han dynasty (25 CE–220 CE), Lingnan became an area in which *zhang* was thought to be endemic. Existing studies formulate the development of the concept of *zhang* as follows: The ceaseless warfare occurring in northern China between the third and sixth centuries impelled a flow of northern immigrants to the south during this period. These immigrants suffered from various unfamiliar disorders in Lingnan, and they used the character for *zhang* as a portmanteau term to denote these.[8]

Along with the increasingly closer connection between Lingnan and the geographical origin of the rampant *zhang* from the third century onward, the early seventh century witnessed the appearance of the first medical treatise that introduced and categorized *zhang*-related disorders in independent sections, rather than discussing them side by side with other disorders. That was *Treatise on the Origins and Symptoms of All Disorders* (Zhubing yuanhou lun, hereafter *Origins and Symptoms*). It was the first such treatise on etiology in China, compiled by the Sui court in 610. In the late sixth century, the founding emperor of the Sui, Wendi (r. 581–604), had ended four hundred years of political division between areas that we now think of as parts of China. After bringing the country back under the control of a single central government, Wendi and the second (and also the last) emperor of the Sui, Yangdi (r. 608–618), extended their unifying efforts to economic and cultural projects, such as dredging the Grand Canal to improve the transportation of goods between northern and southern China. One outcome of these ambitious projects was the completion of *Origins and Symptoms*, whose grand title signals the government's ambition to cover the etiologies of all disorders known at that time. In its section on "symptoms of *zhangqi*," a wide variety of disorders were attributed to *zhangqi* in Lingnan, such as alternating chills and fever, headache, a feeling of fullness in the chest, and a feeling of expansion or bloating in the abdomen.[9] *Origins and Symptoms* provided the foundation of the etiologies and symptoms of *zhang* disorders for all later medical texts.[10]

Given the wide range of phenomena that imperial authors attributed to and categorized under the term *zhang*, recent studies have refrained from translating the term as "malaria" or "miasma."[11] This book likewise does not adopt a singular English translation but instead refers to a *zhang* atmosphere or *zhang* disorders, according to the context. Avoiding translating *zhang* as "malaria" makes sense not only because its meaning varied across narrative contexts but also because retrospectively diagnosing a given historical disorder as a modern disease might kindle a methodological controversy in the field of medical history. Such a retrospective diagnosis presumes that modern disease categories mirror the naturalness or ultimate identity of diseases, representing what medical historians call a "natural-realist approach." Instead, this book applies what scholars call a "historicalist-conceptualist approach," which analyzes concepts of a given disease as historical products shaped by surrounding sociocultural developments.[12]

THE FORMULARY FOR SAVING LIFE IN LINGNAN

Neither Li Qiu's nor Wang Fei's formularies survived as independent texts; instead, they were preserved in partial form in a Yuan-dynasty formulary. After obtaining his *jinshi* degree in 1112, Li traveled extensively during his career as a civil official. In the south, he was appointed to Ying Prefecture (in Guangdong) in 1121, thereafter residing in Cangwu in 1131 and Ji Prefecture (in Jiangxi) in 1134.[13] The court then promoted Li to the rank of "imperial attendant" (*daizhi*) in 1139, and he became the magistrate of Chengdu Prefecture in 1143.[14] With extensive travel experience but no formal training in medicine, Li wrote a formulary that was devoted to far-southern disorders, which came to be known in the Song and Yuan periods as *Treatise on Zhang*, or alternatively *The Formulary for Saving Life in Lingnan* (Lingnan weisheng fang).[15] The fifteenth-century encyclopedia *Great Compendium of the Yongle Era* includes a formulary by Li Qiu but called it *Treatise and Formulary for Preserving Life in Guangnan* (Guangnan shesheng fang lun).[16] Unfortunately, textual evidence regarding this title is too sparse to infer whether it was another name for Li's *Treatise on Zhang* or if Li wrote two formularies on disorders in Lingnan.

Sometime between 1131 and 1139, Zhang Zhiyuan (1090–1147) expanded Li's *Treatise on Zhang*. He obtained his *jinshi* degree in 1121 and served as the magistrate of Guang Prefecture (in Guangdong) between 1138 and 1140.[17] Zhang left no words indicating how he obtained Li's formulary, while describing at length how meticulously he examined Li's medical opinions after receiving the text. He discussed the formulary with a "physician-scholar" (*yishi*), Wang Zijin of Hua Prefecture (in Henan), and tested the formulas collected therein. After confirming their therapeutic efficacy, Zhang composed his own formulary, in which he recorded the etiology of and prescription strategy for *zhang* disorders in Lingnan in a manner similar to what he saw in Li's work. Zhang's expanded version was also named variously, including *Treatise on Zhang, Treatise on Zhang and Intermittent Fever*, and *The Formulary for Saving Life in Lingnan* (Lingnan weisheng fang).

The short time period that passed between the completion of Li Qiu's *Treatise on Zhang* and the completion of Zhang Zhiyuan's work is noteworthy. In the extant *Treatise on Zhang*, Li mentions no plan to publish the formulary. No more than eight years after its completion, however, Zhang produced a follow-up formulary. Such a short interval suggests the considerable likelihood that Li had published or circulated his formulary, at least in manuscript form, among his acquaintances in Lingnan.

Later, Wang Fei, an official whose background is obscure, commented on both Li's and Zhang's versions and also wrote a follow-up formulary, *Instructing the Lost*, between 1139 and 1177. Unfortunately, none of the formularies written by Li, Zhang, or Wang has survived as an independent work. Only three lengthy essays drawn from each are preserved in a Yuan-dynasty formulary that bears the same title: *The Formulary for Saving Life in Lingnan*. Its author, a Buddhist cleric, Jihong, departed from Henan, traveled in Lingnan sometime between 1254 and 1264, moved to Jiangxi in 1265, and resided in Zhejiang between 1272 and 1274. He treated several people and wrote essays about medicine during his travels. He collected his essays on far-southern disorders and parts of other Song officials' formularies into his *Formulary for Saving Life in Lingnan*, writing a preface to this work in 1283.

Drawing on multiple formularies, the Song officials' medical essays that are preserved in the Yuan edition of *The Formulary for Saving Life in Lingnan* can by no means be simplified as northerners' stereotypes of the far south. Some authors were northerners, whereas others actually came from the south. Li Qiu's "place of origin" (*jiguan*) was Bian (at Kaifeng city in Henan), in the north of Song China. In contrast, Zhang Zhiyuan's was Nanjian Prefecture (in Fujian), in the south of Song China. Wang came from Hui Prefecture (in Anhui). Bearing the authors' diverse places of origin in mind, my analysis of the formularies of Li, Zhang, and Wang are based on the three lengthy essays collected in the Yuan edition of *The Formulary for Saving Life in Lingnan*.

FORMULARIES ON LINGNAN
BEFORE THE TWELFTH CENTURY

Medical texts from early China had already associated a number of disorders with Lingnan before Li Qiu and Wang Fei wrote theirs. Nonetheless, it was in the Tang dynasty that a host of formularies devoted to treating disorders endemic to Lingnan first emerged. Those include Wang Fangqing's *Formulary for Lingnan* (Lingnan fang), Zheng Jingxiu's *Treatise and Formulary for Preserving Life in Guangnan in Four Seasons* (Guangnan sishi shesheng fang lun), Li Xuan's *Treatise on Foot Qi in Lingnan* (Lingnan jiaoqi lun), and an anonymous author's *Essential Formulas for Urgent Conditions in Lingnan* (Lingnan jiyao fang).[18] (Wang Fangqing was the commander-in-chief of Guang Prefecture [in Guangdong] sometime between 690 and 694.)[19] Unfortunately, those Tang-era formularies are either lost or remained only as fragments that were preserved in later literature.

While they did not write books, other Tang officials who were appointed to Lingnan recorded and distributed medical formulas for treating disorders there. For example, Liu Zongyuan, who was the regional inspector in Liu Prefecture (in Guangxi) in 815, documented three such formulas and sent them to his friend, Liu Yuxi, who was exiled to Lian Prefecture (in Guangdong) in 815. Liu Yuxi later collected the three formulas into his own formulary, *Passing on Trustworthy Formulas*, and distributed it to his friends. Historians attribute the surge in Lingnan-specific formularies and formulas in the Tang dynasty to the rising medical need created by the increasing number of northern officials and immigrants who shifted to the far south during this period.[20]

The fall of the Tang dynasty in 907 introduced the nearly sixty-year political fragmentation of China known as Five Dynasties and Ten Kingdoms (907–960). Small local states were established and succeeded one another until the Song state conquered them and brought a considerable part of China back under the authority of a single government. After the conquest of Lingnan in 971, the Song emperors and local governments immediately conducted a series of campaigns against perceived unorthodox healing customs in Lingnan, customs that included a preference for "spirit mediums" (*wu*) over physicians, the abandonment of sick relatives, and the cultivation of "*gu*-poisoning" (*gu*).[21] One major means the Song government used across the Lingnan region to promote physicians instead of spirit mediums was to distribute medical texts. This took place at least ten times between the 970s and the 1120s. In 971, Fan Min, the governor of Yong Prefecture (in Guangxi), engraved unspecified formularies on stone stelae on a wall of the government hall.[22] Three years later, the court provided people in Qiong Prefecture (on Hainan Island) unspecified formularies and pharmacological collections.[23] Given that Lingnan was a newly conquered territory, these two policies were highly likely to have been designed to display the authority and presence of the Song state.

In 992, the court distributed a printed version of *The Imperial Grace Formulary* to all prefectures.[24] In the 990s, Chen Yaosou, the fiscal commissioner of the Guangnan West circuit, engraved *A Collection of Effective Formulas* (Jiyan fang) on stone stelae at postal stations in Gui Prefecture (in Guangxi).[25] In 998, the court accepted Chen's suggestion to produce and disseminate "medical formulas and formularies that can preserve life" to prefectures in Lingnan.[26] The court also "gave" (*ci*) *The Imperial Grace Formulary* to Lingnan in 1006.[27] In 1018, the court gave to prefectural offices in Lingnan Zheng Jingxiu's *Treatises on Preserving Life in Guangnan in Four Seasons* and medical formulas that Chen Yaosou collected.[28] An edict in 1051 ordered officials to select formulas for treating epidemics and "*zhang* pestilence" (*zhangli*) from *The Imperial Grace Formulary* to be transcribed on placards at places where epidemics and *zhang* pestilence had occurred.[29] The court in 1072 gave copies of *Treatise on Preserving Life* (Shesheng lun, presumably written by Zheng Jingxiu) and *The Imperial Grace Formulary* to every prefecture in Lingnan.[30]

In addition to the abovementioned ten occasions on which medical texts were distributed in Lingnan, some Song officials stationed there disseminated such texts in their administrative regions without claiming that they wanted to transform local customs perceived as unorthodox. For example, when he was named magistrate of Yu Prefecture (in Guangxi) sometime between 1086 and 1093, He Yujuan wrote *Summary of Preserving and Nurturing Life in Guangnan in Four Seasons* (Guangnan sishi sheyang kuozi) and disseminated the printed edition to the "people" (*ren*) in the prefecture.[31] Lü Wei, an official at the Guangnan West circuit, inscribed the formula for a decoction that could nurture qi on stone stelae that were erected in 1112 in Gui Prefecture (in Guangxi).[32]

The Northern Song officials' involvement in distributing or writing medical texts on far-southern disorders may have resulted from multiple motives, such as a desire to meet their own medical needs or an aspiration to transform and educate locals. Another motive might have involved the military need to prevent Song soldiers in the far-southern frontiers from contracting debilitating disorders. The legendary general and military official Di Qing (1008–1057), once suggested to Emperor Renzong that he order officials in Lingnan to search for elderly people who had been exiled there but remained healthy, learn how they maintained their healthy bodies, and then distribute descriptions of their practices in printed form to soldiers there.[33] Di's suggestion came at a time when the Jiaozhi Ly Kingdom's invasion of Guangxi and the Nong Zhigao rebellion there led the Song state to exert tighter administrative and military control over the area. Following that, Guangxi was considered an important southern frontier until the end of the Southern Song era.[34]

In short, some Tang and Northern Song officials who were assigned to Lingnan wrote about local disorders and their treatments. These writers attributed their work to various purposes, such as meeting their own medical needs, transforming and educating commoners in Lingnan, and saving lives. They also distributed medical treatises in several ways, which included circulating hand-copied manuscripts, engraving remedies on stone steles, and disseminating printed editions. Like their Tang and Song predecessors, Li Qiu and Wang Fei wrote and distributed formularies to save lives in Lingnan.

THE PERCEIVED DEARTH OF RELIABLE MEDICAL TREATISES

Although multiple Tang formularies addressed far-southern disorders and the Song government disseminated many such works in Lingnan, Li Qiu and Wang Fei saw none of those as a reliable treatise for treating endemic disorders in the far south.[35] This perceived absence contrasts with the canonization of Zhang Ji's *Treatise on Cold Damage* that took place in the context of cold damage medicine in Li's day. As we will see, Li's and Wang's formularies and *The Imperial Grace Formulary*—an encyclopedic work that the Song court compiled and then distributed in Lingnan at least four times before Li completed *Treatise on Zhang*—differ in several significant ways with respect to the types of far-southern disorders under discussion, the role of poison or toxicity (*du*) in the etiology of those disorders, and the emphasis on tailoring prescription strategies to individuals' symptomatic and bodily particularities. These differences help to explain why Li and Wang were reluctant to appeal to earlier medical authors as a persuasion strategy but instead proposed their own therapeutic recommendations with the support of the empirical strategy.

One obvious difference between Li's and Wang's formularies, on the one hand, and *The Imperial Grace Formulary*, on the other, concerns the types of far-southern disorders being discussed. *The Imperial Grace Formulary* records three types of disorders that were occurring in Lingnan: "*zhang* poison [bringing in] foot qi" (*zhangdu jiaoqi*), grass *gu*-poisoning (*cao gu shu*), and "mountain *zhang*–intermittent fever" (*shan zhangnüe*).[36] In contrast, Li's and Wang's formularies focused only on *zhang*-related disorders, one of which was "*zhang* and intermittent fever." As their original formularies have survived only partially, it is no longer possible to determine whether the lost texts mentioned other types of far-southern disorders.

A second difference between the three formularies is that the concept of "poison or toxicity" (*du*) is less crucial to the etiology of southern disorders in Li's and Wang's formularies than that for the three types of far-southern disorders listed in *The Imperial Grace Formulary*.[37] *The Imperial Grace Formulary* offers only a brief description of grass *gu*-poisoning, saying that residents of Lingnan and Xiliang often administered it. Once the toxin of grass *gu*-poisoning entered a person's throat, she would feel so much pain that she would rather die.[38]

Gu (often translated as "*gu*-poisoning") is a complex term that signifies either witchcraft or a range of disorders that were often ascribed to venom, insect bites (*chong*), or the practice of using magic to harm others.[39] During the Tang dynasty, *gu*-poisoning was associated with the lower Yangzi area, Fujian, and Lingnan.[40] An edict issued in 1040 reveals the long-standing perception of a connection between *gu*-poisoning and the south in the Song era. The edict prohibited commoners in the southern and western territories of Northern Song China, including Lingnan, from "cultivating" (or "storing," *xu*) poison emitted by snakes or *gu*-poisoning medicines, as well as killing people to worship "bewitching deities" (*yaoshen*).[41] *Gu*-poisoning had also been associated with non-Han ethnic minority groups, such as Miao groups in Lingnan and on the southwest frontier of China.

"*Zhang* poison foot qi" as a subtype of disease first appears in *The Imperial Grace Formulary*, whereas the term "foot qi" (*jiaoqi*) can be traced back to the fourth century. Ge Hong in his *Formulary Kept in One's Sleeve* maintains that foot qi disorders originated in Lingnan and then spread northward to Jiangdong (literally, east of the river, referring to a region east of the lower Yangzi River).[42] As existing scholarship indicates, among the seventy-three categories of disorders in *The Formulary Kept in One's Sleeve*, foot qi is the only one whose region of origin is noted.[43] Ge said that the disease originated in Lingnan and then spread to Jiangdong but did not discuss its etiology. From the fourth century to the Song dynasty, a variety of symptoms were recorded in medical treatises

112 CHAPTER FOUR

under the disease category "foot qi." They included weakness, swelling, painful feet, "an extended and taut chest and abdomen" (*xinfu zhangji*, or inflated abdomen and taut heart), and headaches.[44] These symptoms were all perceived as having originated in the feet and were subsumed by the name "foot qi" (which was occasionally called *jiaoruo*, literally, "foot weakness").

Origins and Symptoms ascribed foot qi to the body's "resonance" (*gan*) with "wind poison" (*fengdu*).[45] Given the low-lying topology of Jiangdong and Lingnan, "the qi of wind and dampness" that arose from the land would easily sicken people and trigger foot qi.[46] The etiology offered in *Origins and Symptoms* was adopted in *The Imperial Grace Formulary*.[47] The authors of the latter identified the low-lying land, dampness, and *zhang* poison as disorder-inducing environmental features of a harmful atmosphere in Jiangdong and Lingnan.

The introduction to "mountain *zhang*–intermittent fever" in *The Imperial Grace Formulary* is almost the same as that in *Origins and Symptoms*, which states that it occurred in Lingnan and the symptoms consisted primarily of alternating chills and fever. This disorder resulted from the "qi of damp poison" (*shi du qi*) in streams and mountain peaks.[48] *Nüe* (intermittent fevers) refers primarily to any type of intermittent chills and fever, which in imperial Chinese medical treatises could be either a systematic disorder or a symptom of such a disorder.[49] *Nüe* could be treated either by pharmacotherapy or religious healing.[50] Following the publication of *Origins and Symptoms*, medical texts discussed *zhang* with *nüe* more frequently.

The centrality of poison is evident in the abovementioned discussion of far-southern disorders in *The Imperial Grace Formulary*, namely, grass *gu*-poisoning practices, *zhang* poison triggering an outbreak of foot qi in Jiangdong and Lingnan, and the qi of damp poison causing mountain *zhang*–intermittent fever. Other examples can be seen in the entry on "zhangqi symptoms" in *Origins and Symptoms*, which associates the occurrence of blue-green grass *zhang* disorders and yellow floss grass *zhang* disorders in Lingnan with "miscellaneous types of poison" (*zadu*) resulting from the warmth there.[51]

In contrast, the concept of poison seldom appears in Li Qiu or Wang Fei's explanations of the occurrence of *zhang* disorders; the two authors described the disorder-inducing environmental features of Lingnan in relatively neutral tones. Li proposed that Lingnan was a "terroir of flame" (*yanfang*) and the land was thin; these two characteristics caused the qi of yang-heat there constantly to "disperse" (*xie*) itself. The term "terroir of flame" served as a reference to the south in general, and sometimes Lingnan specifically, in both historiographical texts and literature.[52] Lingnan occupied low-lying land near the sea; these two features rendered the qi of yin-dampness constantly abundant. The qi of yang-heat and the qi of yin-dampness constantly attacked each other, which gave rise to the syndrome of heat (in my reading, a burning sensation) in the upper body and coldness in the lower body—in Li's views, this was a typical syndrome of "*zhang* disorders" (*zhangji*).[53] On this account, dampness and low-lying land remain relevant as disorder-inducing environmental features, while no reference to poison is made.

Like Li, Wang Fei concentrated on environmental features as disorder-inducing factors without mentioning poison. For instance, he attributed the occurrence of hot *zhang* (one of three types of *zhang* disorders he discussed) to reckless behavior, such as walking in the hot sun during warm seasons without drinking enough water and thus experiencing severe symptoms from the "summer heat." Although the hot climate in Lingnan remained health-threatening, Wang did not employ the concept of poison. He even warned that, although "formularies" (Wang did not specify their titles, calling them only *fangshu*) posited that poison existing between heaven and earth, between water and spring water, and between grass and trees in Lingnan would affect people and caused their disorders, readers should not stick slavishly to this etiology. Wang's warning calls for explicit reflection on the traditional etiology that highlighted poison as a chief cause of disorders in Lingnan. Diverging from the poison-centered explanation, Li and Wang understood disorders in Lingnan differently from the authors of earlier mainstream medical treatises.

The third difference between *The Imperial Grace Formulary* and Li's and Wang's work can be seen in Li's emphasis on a prescription strategy that was tailored to individuals' symptomatic and bodily particularities.[54] *The Imperial Grace Formulary* provides standardized remedies but rarely specifies how readers might modify its medical formulas according to the particular circumstances of the sick. In comparison, Li offered information about prescription strategies for treating a wider range of symptoms and progressions of *zhang* disorders.

These three differences help to explain why Li Qiu and Wang Fei neither recognized earlier formularies as reliable texts for treating *zhang* disorders nor cited them as a persuasion strategy. Instead of advocating for specific medical treatises, Li detailed his success in treating *zhang* disorders in Cangwu, and Wang Fei documented his daily practices that were designed for maintaining health in Lingnan.

DEVELOPING THERAPIES BY TRIAL AND ERROR

Li Qiu used an empirical strategy to prove the trustworthiness of treatments that he developed for addressing *zhang* disorders by delineating the process in which he applied them and attained successful results. His descriptions of his healing success began with his criticism of physicians in Lingnan for failing to notice the obvious connection between the pattern of the external qi there and the specific syndrome of *zhang* disorders (namely, heat in the upper body and coldness in the lower body), thereby prescribing ineffective medicines. According to Li, their ignorance of the true cause of the *zhang* disorders led physicians to mistakenly diagnose a patient's symptoms—being "depleted" (*xu*), "upset" (*fan*), "compressed" (*yu*), or "oppressed" (*men*)—as manifestations of heat inside the body when they were actually symptoms of *zhang* disorders. When treating misdiagnosed heat, those physicians prescribed either medicine to "discharge the exterior condition" (*fabiao*), which in turn damaged the infirm yang qi in their patients' bodies, or drugs that were intended to "disinhibit" (*li*) and "purge" (*xia*) the heat, which in turn exacerbated the coldness in the patient's lower body. Li condemned the physicians because people were dying not from *zhang* pestilence but rather their ineptitude and mistaken prescriptions.[55]

Following his criticism of incompetent physicians, Li described an outbreak of *zhang* pestilence that he witnessed in Cangwu, after which he developed medicinally effective treatments for *zhang* disorders that performed better than the so-called inept physicians' prescriptions. In 1130, an outbreak of *zhang* pestilence was so severe that almost everyone in the families of prominent local officials Wang Jizhi, Zhang Ding, and Ge Tuan died. Li moved to Cangwu the next year and remained there, witnessing countless locals and northern visitors suffering from fatal *zhang* pestilence. Li asked which drugs "the unfortunate" individuals had consumed and discovered that they consisted mainly of ephedra (*mahuang*), bupleurum (*chaihu*), turtle shell (*biejia*), and White Tiger Decoction. Indeed, Li himself contracted the pestilence and became seriously ill in the same year. As shown in the quotation cited at the opening of this chapter, he applied a set of remedies to himself and recovered fully.[56]

During this outbreak of *zhang* pestilence, Li's two servants also fell ill. They experienced "focal distention" (*pi*) and felt stuffed, upset, and restless in their chests. One fainted and another asked for drugs with a cooling quality to refresh and disinhibit his diaphragm and stomach. Li discerned their disorders and then learned that both the servants were actually suffering from heat syndrome in their upper body parts and coldness in their lower ones. He prescribed Decoction of Fresh Ginger and Aconite (Shengjiang Fuzi Tang) rather than drugs with a cooling quality, as the servant requested. He let the decoction cool down first before allowing the servants to consume it. They regained consciousness the next day and said that their chests and diaphragms felt fresh and cool, a sensation associated with cooling drugs, without realizing that it was aconite, a drug thought in pharmacological manuals to be associated with extremely hot qualities, that had brought them relief. The next morning, Li asked them to consume pills of cinnabar when their stomachs were empty, followed by porridge. Next, he applied drugs that were therapeutically effective at "normalizing qi" (*zhengqi*) and "calming the stomach" (*pingwei*). As a result of this series of treatments, the servants recovered fully. After learning about the therapeutic efficacy of these treatments, Li applied the Decoction of Fresh Ginger and Aconite to ten of his acquaintances. All ten were saved.[57]

The sequence in which Li used the set of remedies he prescribed to treat his servants first and then his acquaintances indicates that Li himself was not absolutely certain of the therapeutic efficacy of the remedies. This implies that this application of the decoction to treat *zhang* pestilence was not common in Lingnan, or at least not in Cangwu, in the early 1130s.

After detailing his healing success, Li devoted the second part of his long essay to explaining the mechanism through which the Decoction of Fresh Ginger and Aconite achieved efficacy, as well as giving instructions for prescription strategies for applying other drug remedies in accordance with particular symptoms. For instance, he indicated that if a sick individual's chest was upset and oppressed, the ailing person could consume the cooled decoction; otherwise, in Li's opinion, the efficacy of aconite could manifest too quickly. In addition, Li explained how to apply three other drug remedies to complement the decoction. Unfortunately, none of the specific ingredients in the three remedies collected in *Treatise on Zhang* remain available to us.

Li instructed that the priority for treating *zhang* should be to stabilize the root and normalize the qi of the body. The Decoction of Fresh Ginger and Aconite could achieve this desired therapeutic outcome for most cases of *zhang* disorders. Once the sick person's primary qi was stabilized and restored to a normal condition, the patient could consume "the Ground Powder of the Seven Preciousnesses" (Qibao Cuo San). If physicians could not determine a patient's symptoms or wondered whether the person was suffering from a heat symptom, Jiahe Powders (Jiahe San) provided a suitable alternative.[58] In contrast to the abovementioned prescription strategies, *The Imperial Grace Formulary* merely listed a number of medical formulas in an item-by-item format, explaining little to its readers regarding the sequence that should be followed in choosing and applying them in accordance with the progression of a disorder.

Instructing the Lost begins with an introduction to Wang Fei's medical knowledge and training, which helps to establish the credibility and reliability of the medical opinions that follow. Wang had studied medicine, especially formulas and pulse diagnosis, before moving to Lingnan. He did not specify from whom he learned medicine, a fact that implies that he was self-taught, or at least did not receive training from a master on a regular basis. After arriving in Lingnan, he invited a "senior physician" (or, an elder physician, *laoyi*) in Guilin (in Guangxi) to discuss formularies he had read.

Instructing the Lost then turns to a comparison between Wang's experiences in Lingnan with health environments and disorders recorded in other formularies, elaborating on discrepancies between his experiences and the records. In this comparison, he concurred with Li Qiu's and Zhang Zhiyuan's formularies but was disappointed by their failure to account for the "pulse patterns and breath" (*maixi*) in treating *zhang* disorders. In Wang's view, this omission made it difficult for *zhang* sufferers to use Li's and Zhang's formularies to find formulas that fit their symptoms. It was this concern that moved him to compose *Instructing the Lost*.[59]

In fact, the extant part of Li's and Zhang's *Treatise on Zhang* does briefly mention pulse diagnosis of *zhang* disorders. Li warned his readers that they could not apply decoctions containing aconite when a sick person's eyes turned red and yellow or when their pulse pattern did not indicate the presence of heat syndrome in the upper body and coldness in the lower body. Li then presented his own witness as evidence: when he was in Cangwu, among some one hundred people suffering from *zhang* disorders, only the defense commissioner, Mr. Zheng, presented alternating chills and fever without sweating, and his pulse pattern was "surging and floating." Mr. Zheng thereby took a Minor Bupleurum Decoction (Xiao Chaihu Tang) rather than ones containing aconite, and recovered.[60]

The importance of pulse diagnosis in discerning types of *zhang* disorders in both Li's and Wang's formularies meant that the two authors assumed that their readers knew how to diagnose and distinguish between distinct pulse patterns. Intended for an audience with knowledge of pulse diagnosis, their formularies likely targeted readers who were familiar with medical treatises, not residents of Lingnan, who were often depicted as knowing little about classical medicine. The readership Wang had in mind might have included physicians, medical officials, and civil officials.

After comparing his direct local experience with what he had learned from texts, Wang also deployed an empirical strategy to advocate for maintaining a well-regulated lifestyle as a primary method of preventing disorders in Lingnan. As an official, Wang first resided in Cangwu and then in Liucheng (in Guangxi), Yiyang, and finally Rong Prefecture. Wang claimed that his experiences and observations in these southern regions proved that the local environment was not as lethal as the texts available to him had suggested; for example, mist (which many medical authors deemed a source of disorders in the south) did not actually occur every day but only once every two days. Administrative staff and soldiers suffered disorders caused more by their unregulated lifestyles than by the environment. Wang further shared his routine for maintaining health after his residency in Lingnan. This included the following steps: after arising, a person would consume Powder to Calm the Stomach (Pingwei San) and eat a small portion of porridge; eat breakfast between nine and eleven o'clock in the morning and dinner between three and five o'clock in the afternoon; and, when attending social events, consume alcohol moderately. Wang concluded his long medical essay by noting that "I straightforwardly stated what I heard and saw so as to benefit smart readers to a slight extent."[61] The phrase "heard and saw" (*wenjian*) appears frequently in Song notebooks. In *Instructing the Lost*, the term refers to Wang's personal experience in Lingnan.

MEDICAL STATEMENTS
AND THEIR SOCIAL IMPLICATIONS

In addition to writing formularies, scholar-officials used notebook-style texts to document their experience in Lingnan and to inform medical statements related to that experience. The practice had already spread through notebook-style writings beginning in the late ninth century: scholar-officials verified information pertaining to regional phenomena about which they had previously read and heard and documented their personal experiences in the places in question. The authors of those late ninth-century writings often wrote about Lingnan. In addition to Duan Gonglu's *Northward-Facing Doors*, another work by an official who spent time in Lingnan and recorded his opinions of local disorders and medicinal substances is Liu Xun's *Recording the Extraordinary beyond the Ling Ranges.* In that work, Liu proposes that *zhang* results from Lingnan's mountainous landscape and waterways.[62] The practice of verifying information about regional phenomena and documenting authors' eyewitness experiences in a given region continued well into the twelfth century, extending from medical treatises to notebooks and from travel literature to local gazetteers.[63]

Southern Song authors who wrote down their personal experiences of Lingnan in their notebook-style writings found that the less-structured style was more appropriate for presenting their relatively random thoughts on far-southern medicine, thoughts that were not systematic enough to be composed into a lengthy piece of medical writing or a medical monograph. The prominence of this practice among scholar-officials' writings in the Southern Song era helps not only to justify Li Qiu's and Wang Fei's application of the empirical strategy but also to enhance the evidential value of this strategy.

Regarding the practice of documenting authors' experiences in Lingnan and related medical opinions during the Southern Song era, one case in point is "Ten Talks about the Lingbiao area" (*Lingbiao shishuo,* hereafter "Ten Talks"), a long essay preserved by the Yuan edition of *Formulary for Saving Life in Lingnan.* The author of this essay, Zhang Jie, was the administrative assistant of the fiscal commission of the Guangnan East circuit between 1133 and 1134 and was promoted to vice fiscal commissioner of the same circuit between 1137 and 1139. "Ten Talks" consists of ten entries, each of which covers a topic related to maintaining health in Lingnan, including remarks on the local habit of eating betel nuts and consuming alcoholic drinks to avoid contracting *zhang,* descriptions of potentially debilitating environmental features, the etiology of *zhang* disorders, and advice on an appropriate lifestyle for living in Lingnan. In one of the ten talks, Zhang clearly uses a first-person pronoun that means "your humble servant" (*pu*). In addition, the vivid descriptions of various aspects of Lingnan and his comments on them reinforce the impression that he was drawing to some degree on his own experiences and observations there.

The entry of "Ten Talks" that best illustrates Zhang's interest in arguing about healing affairs in Lingnan is one in which he argues against the notion that consuming alcohol could prevent *zhang,* saying that a pharmacological manual recorded the notion. Although he did not specify its title, Song authors, when disagreeing with the idea of consuming alcohol to prevent *zhang,* often referred to a story in Tao Hongjing's *Collected Annotations.* The story reads as follows: Once upon a time, three people encountered mist when traveling in the morning. Later, one was fine, another became ill, and the third one died. Before setting off, the healthy one had consumed alcoholic drinks, the sick one had consumed porridge, and the dead one had eaten nothing. Tao Hongjing suggested that the healthy one was fine because of the "propensity" (*shi*) of alcohol to repel malicious substances.[64] Even though the story did not indicate whether the mist was a *zhang* atmosphere or not, the Song authors frequently mentioned this story when refuting the notion that drinking alcohol could prevent *zhang*.[65] Disagreeing with this notion, Zhang proposed that it was indulgence in drinking that actually caused people to suffer *zhang*, claiming that "the earth of the south is summer heat and dampness. If one indulges in drinking alcohol, then one usually is struck by the poison of summer heat."[66] Zhang's word of caution reminds us of Wang Fei's abovementioned daily routine for maintaining health.

Fan Chengda was another avid participant in the scholarly trend whereby authors verified putative regional characteristics, documented their experiences, and registered their medical opinions regarding illnesses in Lingnan. Fan was a magistrate in Jingjiang Prefecture (in Guangxi) between 1172 and 1175, after which, in 1175, he was assigned to Chengdu (in Sichuan). On his way there, he recalled his times in Jingjiang Prefecture and composed *Treatises of the Supervision and Guardian of the Cinnamon Sea* (Guihai yuheng zhi, hereafter *Cinnamon Sea*). *Cinnamon Sea* comprises information that Fan collected about the Guangnan East circuit and his experience in this region. He divided it thematically into thirteen chapters, discussing relevant topics in an entry-by-entry format in each.[67] Fan's chapters and entries cover a broad range of topics, such as precipice-grottoes, metals, stones, aromatics, alcoholic drinks, birds, flowers, fruits, and ethnic-minority groups living there.

In one entry on *zhang* in a chapter on miscellaneous items, Fan addressed its occurrence of and remedies for it. He noted that the south of Guilin (in Guangxi) was home to *zhang*, which resulted from mountain mists and watery poisons together with foul gas emitted by wild grasses and a steamy swelter from lush vegetation. Victims of the *zhang* atmosphere looked like they had contracted intermittent fever. Although there were many extant treatments, aconite was usually used in urgent cases while "Priceless Qi-Correcting Powder" (Buhuan Jin Zhengqi San) was used in less urgent cases.[68] Fan did not specify who used aconite or the powder, the ingredients the powder contained, or how to make it. That he mentioned only the powder's name without providing any information about its composition or manufacture suggests that Fan either

120 CHAPTER FOUR

assumed that readers already knew about it or assumed that they would consult other sources when seeking to treat *zhang*-caused intermittent fever.

Apart from those who wrote entirely about Lingnan, other Southern Song authors recorded their experiences of and medical opinions about the area as a part of their notebooks on a wider range of topics, which is exemplified by *Jade Dew in the Crane Forest* (Helin yulu) by Luo Dajing (1196–1242?, *jinshi* 1226), who once was the judicial administrator of Rong Prefecture. In an entry on betel nuts, Luo first indicates that locals in Lingnan ate them as an alternative to drinking tea, believing that this could help them "resist *zhang*" (*yuzhang*), thus preventing adverse reactions to a *zhang* atmosphere or suffering from *zhang* disorders. He recalled that when he arrived in Lingnan, he could not bear to eat betel nuts. After staying a while, though, he learned to eat a small number of them. After a year there, he found that he could not live without them for a single day. Luo then proposed four benefits of betel nuts, including facilitating digestion.[69]

Among the Southern Song notebooks that contained authors' experiences of and medical opinions about Lingnan, *Vicarious Replies from beyond the Ling Ranges* (Lingwai daida, hereafter *Vicarious Replies*) is particularly noteworthy because its author, Zhou Qufei (ca. 1134–?), reproduced part of Wang Fei's *Instructing the Lost*. Zhou, originally from Yongjia (in Zhejiang), lived more of his life as a northerner than as a resident of Lingnan. He earned his *jinshi* degree in 1163 but never rose into higher echelons of bureaucratic systems. He served as a low-ranking official in Qin Prefecture and Jingjiang Prefecture (both in Guangxi), from approximately 1172 to 1178.[70] He was also an acquaintance of Fan Chengda in Guilin. After moving northward from Lingnan, he compiled *Vicarious Replies* in 1178. Zhou notes in his preface that when writing *Vicarious Replies*, he drew from his experience and observations in Lingnan, entries in *Cinnamon Sea*, and other texts that he did not specify.[71] In *Vicarious Replies*, Zhou neither mentions Wang Fei by name nor addresses his formulary by its title. In one entry on *zhang*, however, Zhou repeats Wang's description of three types of *zhang* disorders in an identical manner.

To show the resemblance between Zhou Qufei's entry on *zhang* and Wang Fei's discussion of *zhang* disorders, I introduce Wang's discussion first and compare it with Zhou's entry. Wang began his discussion by noting the etiology of *zhang* disorders recorded in "statements of formularies that [he] now reads." It ran as follows: the qi of heaven in the south was warm, and the qi of earth was compressed and steaming. The yin was constantly "closed" (*bi*), and the yang was emitted and dispersed. Grass, woods, and water in the south all received malicious qi. Living in such a debilitating environment, inhabitants gradually developed infirm primordial qi, which resonated with the malicious qi, and thus suffered from *zhang* disorders. Those who suffered only mildly would experience symptoms that included hot and cold flushes, which was similar to suffering intermittent fevers. This type of *zhang* disorder was called "cold *zhang*." Those who suffered more seriously would experience heat (burning sensations) inside the body that felt like they were lying on burning charcoal. This type was called "hot *zhang*." Those suffering from the most serious *zhang* disorders would become mute for unknown reasons, thereupon leading to its being known as "muteness-causing *zhang*" (*yazhang*). Immediately after describing the three types of *zhang* disorders, Wang commented that "this is what formularies say; however, in my shallow view, what is called muteness-causing *zhang* is voice-loss cold damage disorders. Isn't it?"[72] This comment refers to the analogy as Wang's innovative notion. In comparison, in *Vicarious Replies*, Zhou Qufei repeated Wang's summary of the etiology and three disorder types almost verbatim. More importantly, Zhou also proposed that treatments for voice-loss cold damage disorders could be applied to treat muteness-causing *zhang*, a therapeutic recommendation clearly inspired by Wang's analogy.[73]

Zhou's use of Wang's *Instructing the Lost* indicates the short time over which that medical treatise circulated among officials who were stationed in Guangxi. This is reminiscent of the short time it took for Zhang Zhiyuan to review Li Qiu's *Treatise on Zhang* as well as for Wang to review Li's and Zhang's formularies. The rapid circulation of Li's, Zhang's, and Wang's formularies among officials in Lingnan collectively attests to a case, that is, that other contemporaneous civil officials serving in Lingnan constituted an important readership of medical texts that Southern Song officials there wrote about the treatment of far-southern disorders. Those civil officials had not, for the most part, received expert medical training but were familiar with medicine through reading. They were likewise articulate in their views of healing affairs in Lingnan, either in their medical works or in their notebook-style writings.

By relocating the contents of Wang's formulary to his own notebook, Zhou expanded the social implications of medical knowledge from treating the sick to demonstrating an author's erudition. He lived at a time when the number of less politically established scholar-officials and the number of notebooks both rose precipitously. Those scholar-officials had either attempted but failed to pass the civil service examination or had passed but had struggled in low echelons of bureaucratic systems throughout their lives. They acquired knowledge on assorted topics through hands-on experience or through traveling as examinees or civil servants. The characteristic features of a notebook—its wide topical coverage and item-to-item presentation in a casual and less-structured organization—enabled those politically underachieving scholar-officials to share their knowledge on various subjects. By compiling such a wide array of knowledge in their notebooks, they were signaling their erudition and building up their sense of themselves as intellectual elites, despite their less than fully successful political careers.[74]

Zhou Qufei's *Vicarious Replies* epitomizes this Southern Song trend. In his preface, Zhou claims that he wrote it in part because "I am tired of [being asked about things in Lingnan] at social occasions. If someone asks me these questions again, I can use this text instead."[75] The title also signals this purpose. The numerous questions that Zhou's relatives and acquaintances asked, even if he exaggerated somewhat, indicates the high level of curiosity about Lingnan that was common among scholar-officials and laypersons. Such curiosity also suggests that having knowledge of this remote and exotic place had a positive impact on a scholar-official's popularity at social occasions, which occupied a significant portion of their lives in the Song era. They frequently gathered with friends and colleagues, held banquets to welcome newly arrived officials, and attended farewell parties for those whom the court assigned to other locations. At such occasions, contributing novel conversational material was a critical means by which a scholar-official, especially a low-ranking one like Zhou, could display his erudition and enhance his social and cultural fame.[76]

Displaying one's erudition had more practical social implications for low-ranking officials, like Zhou, in the Southern Song era than it did in the Northern Song. We have seen in chapter 2 how Kou Zongshi extended the social functions of a medical treatise by submitting his *Elucidating the Meaning* to the throne in 1116 for possible bureaucratic promotion. Sixty years after Kou's submission, in Zhou's day, low-ranking officials encountered fewer opportunities to move upward through the echelons of bureaucratic systems. The increasingly higher number of candidates in the Southern Song period led to a highly competitive examination. Even though a fortunate few did pass and hence gained the qualifications for entering officialdom, they soon encountered new challenges along their career paths.

Often beginning as "low-level executory officials" (*xuanren*), when seeking promotion to the status of "high-level administrative official" (*jingguan*), applicants needed to assemble portfolios of recommendation letters from five sponsors whose bureaucratic rankings were higher than theirs. The number of letters that each sponsor could write in a given year was limited, depending on his bureaucratic rank.[77] In addition to this limit, a shortage of bureaucratic positions made career advancement more challenging.[78] It was thus crucial for low-level executory officials to maintain and extend their personal networks to acquire the coveted letters. Exhibiting their erudition, gaining popularity at social occasions, and enhancing their cultural and social fame would all help them build networks that could facilitate their advancement. In this regard, having knowledge of medicines as well as exotic Lingnan provided practical social advantages for those marginal officials.

COLD DAMAGE MEDICINE IN THE HOT SOUTH

In addition to employing the empirical strategy, Li Qiu's and Wang Fei's formularies both resemble Southern Song notebook-style writings in another important respect: their shared concern with the applicability of cold damage medicines to Lingnan. This indicates the tighter intertextual space that was emerging between medical literature and notebook-style writings in the Southern Song era.[79] It additionally offers us a glimpse into scholar-officials' uncertainty when applying relatively northern classical medicines to the far south, which contrasts starkly with the assertiveness underlying the Song government's campaign to promote medicine in this region. The contrast reveals practical difficulties in integrating the far south into the "civilized" Chinese empire.[80]

The concern with the applicability of cold damage medicine in Lingnan had already appeared in the seventh century; however, since the Song dynasty came to power, particularly since the twelfth century, it became increasingly pronounced as more authors of nonmedical literature voiced the same concern. The rising urgency of this issue parallels the boost in cold damage medicine in the Song era. Existing scholarship reflects this interest in such medicine by examining predominantly medical texts that refer to cold damage disorders in their titles. In this section, by shifting attention to formularies on Lingnan and notebooks, I reveal the much wider scope of the influences of cold damage medicine on Song-dynasty medicine than existing scholarship has hitherto observed.

The textual evidence for the expansion of cold damage medicine to treatments of disorders in Lingnan can be traced to the early seventh-century *Origins and Symptoms.* This treatise suggests that cold damage medicine was extendable to *zhang* disorders in Lingnan, given that the transmission of *zhang* manifestations through the bodily "channels" (*jing*) and "links" (*luo*) in a patient's body were almost the same as those posited for cold damage disorders north of the Ling ranges. Nevertheless, because of warm seasonal qi in Lingnan, when treating *zhangqi* there, physicians were expected to use drugs of a colder quality than those used to treat cold damage disorders north of the Ling ranges. In a similar vein, drugs with a hot quality that were applied to treat *zhang* disorders in Lingnan should have involved lower doses than those advised for treating cold damage disorders.[81]

The caution regarding regional styles expressed in *Origins and Symptoms* has ancient roots. At least as early as the Han dynasty, the notion already existed that regional differences in diet, climate, and the quality of the land caused inhabitants in separate regions to possess different bodily constitutions and required correspondingly tailored treatments. Although it was implicit, the ancient medical classic *Basic Questions* expressed this notion as well. It addressed regional therapeutic styles in a section entitled "On Different Methods Being Appropriate for Different Directions," which declares that the varying skin patterns of inhabitants in five directions (i.e., east, west, north, south, and center) required matching treatments.[82]

In the Song dynasty, one view that radically challenged the notion of applying cold damage medicine to treatments for *zhang* emerged in a privately compiled formulary, *Discussions on Cold Damage and General Disorders.* Its author, Pang Anshi, was a famous physician and friends with two leading literary figures, Su Shi and Huang Tingjian, in the late eleventh century. Both Su and Huang praised this formulary highly and planned to print it. Eventually, in 1113, an unknown publisher printed the formulary. The first section covers models for diagnosing and prescribing medicine for cold damage disorders, which laid out the theoretical foundation for the rest of his formulary. In that section, Pang claims that "the south is a place where there is no frost and snow, and people there are not being struck by cold qi. The qi of land is not stored. Types of insects emit poison. Mountain mist and *zhang* atmosphere occurred intermittently."[83] Pang thereby notes that disorders endemic in the south require treatments different from those for cold qi–inducing disorders.[84] Although he did not specify the names of any of the southern places to which he referred in making this claim, their characteristics in the quotation all are reminiscent of Lingnan. Pang was registered as having come from Qi Prefecture (in Hubei), being active around this area, and leaving no textual evidence, which suggests that he had been to Lingnan in person.[85] If this were the case, his statement could be viewed as a northern physician's imagining of the far south, where environmental features were very different from those in the center of China and required correspondingly different remedies.

Apart from Pang's remarks, few Northern Song observations about the relationship between cold damage disorders and *zhang* in Lingnan have come down to us. However, Southern Song authors left us additional, more informative, sources of their views regarding the applicability of cold damage medicine to Lingnan. For instance, Chao Gongwu, the famous bibliographer, expressed a view that was similar to Pang's. Chao obtained his *jinshi* degree in 1132, resided in Sichuan for many years, and never visited Lingnan. In his grand bibliographical text, *Memoirs of Reading in the Jun Studio*, he commented that Zhang Ji's *Treatise on Cold Damage* "contains drugs only for healing disorders in the north but was missing treatments for southern disorders."[86]

Although the notion of regionally tailored therapies had already emerged in the Han dynasty, Chinese authors in the twelfth century took this idea a step further by describing how the application of specific drugs should be adapted to the perceived particularities of a given locality, as we shall see regarding Li Qiu's formulary. While not explicitly denying the applicability of cold damage medicine to Lingnan, Li Qiu and Zhang Zhiyuan both adopted cautious attitudes toward the idea. Li criticized what he saw as inept physicians for applying ephedra, bupleurum, or a White Tiger Decoction, which were ingredients or drug therapies more typically used to treat cold damage disorders, as treatments for *zhang* disorders. Echoing Li's criticism of these treatments, Zhang complained that they failed to discern any specific syndromes associated with *zhang* disorders that resulted from Lingnan's environmental features. Consequently, they mistakenly applied "methods of treating wind damage and cold damage disorders in the north," prescribing drugs that cause "sweating" (*han*) and "purging" (*xia*) of the sick, thus losing the lives of "five to six patients out of ten."[87]

Li's and Zhang's criticisms of incompetent physicians in Lingnan emerged during a period when warfare between the Song and Jin states raged continuously across the middle and lower reaches of the Yellow River and the area south of the Huai River in the early to mid-eleventh century. The warfare drove a stream of migrants southward to Lingnan. Some of the physicians Li and Zhang criticized may have recently immigrated from the north, as a result applying cold damage medicine that was prominent in the north to treat the sick in Lingnan. An account supporting this scenario comes from Zhang Jie's "Ten Talks," in which he described "northern physicians" (*beiyi*) arriving in Lingnan and applying a Major Bupleurum Decoction to treat hot *zhang* disorders. As Zhang Jie commented, only those whose fundamental qi was vigorous and replete could bear the effects of the decoction; locals who had consumed betel nuts over a long period of time had already depleted the qi of their organs and thus often could not tolerate drugs with cold quality (such as bupleurum). Zhang did not explain why such northern physicians traveled to Lingnan in the 1130s, a period when he lived in Lingnan, but it seems possible that they were war-weary immigrants.[88]

After the 1130s, scholar-officials expressed a wider variety of views regarding the applicability of cold damage medicine to Lingnan. Wang Fei believed that whether such medicine was applicable varied across distinct types of *zhang* disorders. He claimed that muteness-causing *zhang* was actually a case of losing one's voice as a result of cold damage disorders and being struck by wind. This explanation reflects Wang's efforts to account for *zhang* disorders by drawing on intellectual sources associated with cold damage medicine.

Some Southern Song scholar-officials endeavored to understand *zhang* disorders through language drawn from cold damage medicine. This endeavor is best seen in their explanation of the "picking-grass-seeds" (*tiao caozi*) technique, a set of therapies that locals in Lingnan used to treat *zhang* disorders. Such an explanation appears in a lengthy essay of the Yuan edition of *Formulary for Saving Life in Lingnan*, which is entitled "Wang Nanrong's Discussion on Remedies and Pulse Diagnosis of Cold and Hot *Zhang* Disorders." Modern scholars have long suspected that the Wang Nanrong named as the author of the essay was actually Wang Fei, considering that the character expressing Wang Fei's surname could easily be mistaken as the character that expresses Wang Nanrong's surname and that Wang Fei was the magistrate of Nanrong (i.e., Rong Prefecture) when composing *Instructing the Lost*. In other words, the name "Wang Nanrong" is highly likely to be an admixture of Wang Fei's surname (but with the wrong character) and the place name where Wang Fei completed his formulary. "Grass seeds" (*caozi*) was a local term used in Lingnan in reference to hot and cold epidemics.[89] "Picking grass seeds" then could mean combatting hot and cold epidemics via therapies that involve the use of needles.

Wang Nanrong (or Wang Fei) identified picking grass seeds as the only method for treating hot *zhang* disorders. This method went as follows: When a person suffered from hot *zhang* for more than one to two days, local healing practitioners used needles to prick the middle of the inside part of the sick person's upper and lower lips, wiping the blood off their hands and tongue with leaves of *chu* trees, which belonged to the mulberry tree family. The sick person was then required to stand with his heels together. The practitioner would prick the standing patient's blue vessels on the back of his heels, letting the blood out. After this procedure, the sick person would consume "blue-green wormwood herb" (*qinghao*) with water.[90]

The picking-grass-seeds technique differed remarkably from therapies, such as drug remedies, moxibustion, and acupuncture, that scholarly elites often encountered in medical genres. Regardless, Wang endeavored to explain the therapeutic mechanism underlying this technique via the language of cold damage medicine. He declared that pricking a person suffering from hot *zhang* and letting his blood out actually complied with the therapeutic principle of inducing perspiration. In his view, hot *zhang* disorders were manifestations of "major yang" (*taiyang*) cold damage disorders. After the sick person's major yang area became disordered for three days, his "yang brightness" (*yangming*) area became disordered as well. It was believed to be through the upper and lower lips that the stomach channel of yang brightness passes, while the backs of the heels was where the bladder channel of major yang passes. This was why pricking an ailing person's upper and lower lips and heels could treat the disordered major yang and yang brightness areas. Wang commented that the needling of "southerners" (*nanren*) thus tacitly was consistent with the principle of treating the manifestation of major yang cold damage disorders.[91]

By interpreting a local healing technique using medical language drawn from cold damage medicine, Wang exhibited a relatively positive attitude toward the technique. One contrast to this is found in Fan Chengda's comments on the picking-grass-seeds technique in *Cinnamon Sea*, where he remarked that it had no healing effects and the sick still needed to consume drugs. Wang's interpretation demonstrates a more neutral, Sinocentric perspective on far-southern residents' healing practices than earlier and contemporaneous scholar-officials had been accustomed to expressing.

Although Wang attempted to rationalize the picking-grass-seeds technique by extending cold damage medicine to *zhang* in Lingnan, he nevertheless admitted the limitations of this practice. For instance, for a dying man suffering from hot *zhang* that had penetrated deep into the interior of his body, one therapy suggested was to prick his penis. After describing this, Wang wrote that

"I personally consider" (*qieyi*) that the penis was connected internally to the five visceral systems, and thus pricking it "perhaps" (*huo*) would remove the sick person's interior heat.[92] The phrases "I personally consider" and "perhaps" together suggest Wang's uncertainty about the healing mechanism, which went beyond the scope of his knowledge but nonetheless he deemed worthy of recording as a local therapy.

Zhou Qufei in *Vicarious Replies* likewise talks about the applicability of cold damage medicine in Lingnan. Nevertheless, some of his accounts actually draw from others' formularies. Zhou not only used Wang Fei's equation of muteness-causing *zhang* and voice-loss cold damage disorders without crediting the source, but he also nearly copied the abovementioned description by Wang Nanrong and his explanation of the "picking-grass-seeds" technique. Here again we see how Zhou transformed medical knowledge that was written primarily for healing purposes into knowledge that he used to support his conversational skills and signal his erudition.

Apart from the uncredited use of Wang Fei's and Wang Nanrong's formularies, Zhou also wrote that, in the south, all disorders were called *zhang*; their "reality" (*shi*) was similar to that of cold damage disorders occurring in "central prefectures" (*zhongzhou*) of China. Without clarifying this statement, especially his reference to "reality" and "central prefectures," Zhou explained the etiology of *zhang* and distinguished three types (i.e., Wang Fei's opinions on cold *zhang*, hot *zhang*, and muteness-causing *zhang*). After proposing that treatments for cold damage disorders could be applied to treat hot *zhang* and muteness-causing *zhang*, Zhou reminded his readers that there were still differences between *zhang* and cold damage disorders: "For treating *zhang*, one cannot simply apply drugs used for cold damage disorders occurring in the central prefectures. If one merely sees the sick suffering from heat severely, he then applies the sort of drugs such as 'the crude form of sodium surface' [*poxiao*] and 'rhubarb root' to purge the heat. If the inherited bodily constitution is weak, the sick immediately falls into crisis."[93] Zhou disagreed with a simplistic application of drugs that were used for cold damage disorders in "central prefectures" to treat *zhang* in Lingnan. He warned that physicians merely noticed heat as a symptom of *zhang* disorders and accordingly applied the crude form of sodium surface and rhubarb, two drugs with a cold quality. Overall, like Wang Fei's stance on expanding cold damage medicine to *zhang* disorders, Zhou Qufei's can be summarized as follows: because of the similar essentials associated with these two categories of disorders, the expansion was feasible but had to be conducted with caution and account for sick people's individual bodily constitutions.

THE EMPIRICAL STRATEGY in Li Qiu's and Wang Fei's formularies was based largely on two factors. First, the two authors observed a dearth of reliable medical treatises pertaining to far-southern disorders. On the one hand, since the Tang dynasty, medical authors—including officials in Lingnan—had written multiple treatises devoted to treating these disorders. The Northern Song government actively disseminated medical texts to Lingnan, and local officials engraved formulas on stone stelae. On the other hand, despite the ample number of privately composed and state-disseminated medical treatises, Li and Wang did not find any of them canonical or exemplary for the treatment of *zhang* disorders. Their reluctance to endorse those treatises may reflect distinct understandings of far-southern disorders presented in their formularies and in the earlier works. In the absence of authoritative medical treatises and given a shortage of competent physicians in Lingnan, Li and Wang proposed their preventive and therapeutic recommendations for *zhang* disorders and maintaining health there. The two sought to render their opinions more authoritative by describing in detail their relevant practices and sharing their observations of the practice of medicine in Lingnan.

Another factor that encouraged Li and Wang to rely on the empirical strategy was scholar-officials' long-standing practice of narrating their personal observations of putatively regional phenomena. Since the late ninth century, they had demonstrated a strong interest in verifying information regarding regional particularities about which they read and heard. This interest became more salient in the twelfth century, proliferating across medical texts, notebooks, travel literature, and local gazetteers. Among all the places that had been subjected to scholar-officials' personal inspections, Lingnan, as a remote, untamed area that was dramatically different from the heartland of Chinese civilization, fascinated them. The proliferation of authors' experiences of and medical opinions about Lingnan in the nonmedical literature helped to warrant Li's and Wang's extensive use of the empirical strategy in their formularies.

The twelfth century witnessed not only the greater prevalence of the practice of documenting authors' local experiences but also the emergence of a tighter intertextual space between authors of formularies on Lingnan and notebook writers. This is evident in their shared concerns about the applicability of cold damage medicines in that area. In the early seventh century, medical authors voiced these concerns. Beginning in the twelfth century, notebook authors participated in discussions regarding them, which reflected a heightened awareness of the importance of treating *zhang* disorders in accordance with environmental features and the bodily particularities of sick people in Lingnan. The Song authors' opinions varied considerably, as they disagreed about how and to what degree cold damage medicine could be applied to the etiology and treatment of *zhang* disorders. The variety of opinions regarding Lingnan contrasted starkly with the Northern Song government's active and assertive policies that promoted the expansion of classical medicine to the region. This gap between the political realm, where officials assertively promoted classical medicine as a matter of policy, and local medical practices, where trial-and-error approaches and uncertainty governed the pursuit of effective treatments, reveals the tension between the standardized remedies that the government offered and individualized prescription strategies considered more regionally appropriate. This tension only intensified in subsequent centuries. In the sixteenth century, for example, tailoring prescriptions to individuals and specific circumstances became an essential skill among scholar-physicians as well as a staple narrative theme in the new "medical case statements" genre.

Conclusion

THE EMPIRICAL STRATEGY on which this book has focused appeared in medical literature in the fifth century, became more elaborate in the late ninth century, and rose in salience during the Song dynasty, especially after the eleventh century. It by no means developed along a linear trajectory. The rise of the empirical strategy can be attributed to both individual authorial agendas and broader societal changes in publishing and epistemic cultures that took place between the ninth and twelfth centuries. Beginning in the late ninth century, increasing numbers of authors came to emphasize the importance of establishing the veracity of the information they recorded and disseminated. This included witnessing successful outcomes of formulas, describing the historical contexts in which a poem was composed or circulated, and empirically verifying putative regional phenomena (especially those in the Lingnan region). Such emphases grew apace in the Song era.

Although most Song medical authors did not attribute their inspiration for this new emphasis to their ninth-century predecessors, it is hard to ignore similarities in the great stress that the two groups of authors laid on confirming the veracity of the information they distributed. The burgeoning phenomenon that began in the late ninth century signaled three profound changes in epistemic cultures: greater acceptance of knowledge acquired through hands-on experience as worthy of documentation, the greater presence and epistemic autonomy of individual authors, and the related enhanced intellectual value of the reliability of a given text. Modern scholars have focused specifically on the Song dynasty's contributions to the development of these three trends. But those innovations were not entirely the work of Song authors. Rather, they were continuous with developments that began in the late ninth century and became widely expressed in the Song dynasty.

The abovementioned trends in epistemic cultures in middle-period China appeared in both medical and nonmedical writings, the latter of which included notebooks, travel accounts, and inventories of things. Medical literature in this era engaged in a close intertextual dialogue with nonmedical writings, particularly with notebooks. That is, medical authors could, and often did, comment on medical opinions that had been expressed originally in nonmedical writings, and authors of nonmedical writings often cited and commented on medical treatises. There was no clear boundary between knowledge to be recorded and discussed in medical literature and similar knowledge appearing in nonmedical writings. In combination, this close intertextual dialogue and the absence of a clear boundary render it difficult to gauge the extent to which those nonmedical writings influenced the rise of the empirical strategy in medical literature. At best we can say that the proliferation of this strategy was a function of these broader changes in epistemic cultures, and its prominence in turn enhanced the visibility of these trends.

In addition to these new trends in epistemic cultures during middle-period China, another significant factor contributing to the rise of the empirical strategy in medical literature during the Song period was the new environment surrounding medical publications and learning that emerged in this era. The Song dynasty witnessed prodigious growth in medical text publishing, which resulted in no small part from the Northern Song imperial court's unprecedented sponsorship of the dissemination of medical knowledge and a trend among the literati toward distributing medical texts for the public good. The publishing boom meant greater availability of and access to such texts, therefore expanding the types and numbers of readers interested in medical treatments, a critical mass of whom was unknown to those authors. To convince those readers that their writings were reliable, many of the authors related scenarios in which they empirically verified putative regional phenomena and a given remedy reached a successful outcome. Those narrative accounts worked primarily to affirm the historical factuality of a remedy's efficacy. Some authors (such as Shen Kuo) assumed that their accounts could additionally give lay readers—those who could read medical texts but were unable to customize treatments on their own—clues for matching a sick person's specific symptoms with a given remedy. The empirical strategy thereby helped authors present themselves as benevolent and reliable knowledge distributors.

Meanwhile, the Song dynasty saw increasingly intensified intertextual debates. Readers showed keen interest in comparing and commenting on various medical claims that their contemporaries had written. This interest depended on the simultaneous accessibility of numerous readily available medical texts, an abundance made possible by the expanding public attainability of such literature during this period. Some readers even composed new medical texts containing their own comments, intensifying intertextual debates in which they engaged with other Song authors. To win these debates, some authors (such as Kou Zongshi, Xu Shuwei, and Wang Fei) turned to an empirical strategy.

THE EMPIRICAL STRATEGY IN THE SOUTHERN SONG ERA

In the Southern Song era, the growing visibility of the empirical strategy in medical literature went hand in hand with the wider spread of print technology, as this period witnessed the printing of treatises at unprecedented rates. Among the published treatises, the empirical strategy was used principally to attest to the veracity of events that authors related.

In Southern Song accounts of pharmacological knowledge, authors often used the empirical strategy to verify the efficacy of local medicinal substances and healing practices. This strategy appeared widely in medical and nonmedical literature, such as pharmacological manuals, notebooks, and travel accounts. Apart from verifying textual claims, some authors began recording local medicines that they witnessed, and then compiled those records into independent books. One example of this new practice is *Materia Medica on Lüchan Rocks* (Lüchan yan bencao, 1220, hereafter *Lüchan Rocks*), the earliest extant pharmacological manual in China that was devoted to introducing medicinal substances originating from a specific and narrow geographic region. Its author, Wang Jie, presumably served in the inner court of Ling'an (in Hangzhou city, Zhejiang) during the Qinyuan regime (1195–1201). Wang stressed that all of the some two-hundred medicinal substances that *Lüchan Rocks* recorded were herbs that grew locally, near where he lived on the west slope of Ciyun Mountain (in Zhejiang, near West Lake), and which he observed and used.[1] For instance, in an entry on "bee grass" (*mifeng cao*), Wang noted that his gardener once let him smell the grass's leaves, and he thought it smelled like honey. This led Wang to conclude that this was why it was called bee grass.[2] *Lüchan Rocks* even included illustrations that Wang drew of each of the herbs that he recorded.

In Southern Song formularies, the primary goal in using the empirical strategy was to attest to the historical factuality of a remedy's therapeutic efficacy. Authors often documented informants' names, occupations, and social relations (such as recording that a person lived in the author's home county or was the author's relative). For instance, Hong Zun (1120–1174), in his *Mr. Hong's Collection of Effective Formulas* (Hongshi jiyan fang, 1170), documented the source of his information, indicating the efficacy of almost every remedy he recorded. Such sources typically included his, his relatives,' or his acquaintances' experience applying remedies to achieve the desired efficacy, as well as their witnessing of a successful outcome of a given remedy. For example, Hong remarked that when he was in Poyang (in Jiangxi), a person had seemingly died of drowning, but the remedy brought the victim back to consciousness.[3] In an entry about using moxibustion, Hong indicated that it was "Guo Tinggui, the administrator of a district," who had transmitted this method to him. Hong described how Guo witnessed its miraculous efficacy.[4] In many entries, Hong meticulously noted each informant's name, bureaucratic position, and geographical location, demonstrating his heedfulness of the need to prove the historical factuality of his records.[5]

Two other exemplary formularies whose authors used the empirical strategy to prove that they were historically factual and therapeutically effective are Ye Dalian's *Mr. Ye's Collection of Effective Formulas* (Yeshi luyan fang, 1186) and Wei Xian's *Mr. Wei's Family Collection of Formulas* (Weishi jiacang fang, 1227). Ye, who was a low-ranking official, carved his formulary into woodblocks in 1186. In its preface, Ye said that that the formulas collected in the treatise came from "those his previous generations passed down" and "those he favored to use in the ordinary day"; as for medical formulas that "I had seen no one using, I applied them but did not see their efficacy, and those I doubted and dared not rashly apply, all of such formulas I dare not transmit to others."[6] Wei remarked that his formulary collected 1,151 formulas, all based on remedies that he, his father, and his grandfather used and found effective.[7] Notably, Wei Xian, Ye Dalian, and Hong Zun all expressed their intentions to print their formularies to extend the scope of their works' circulation.

The emphasis on the historical factuality of recorded events and authors' keen attention to noting information sources prevailed in Southern Song notebooks, among which Hong Mai's *Record of the Listener* is emblematic. *Record of the Listener* was widely printed across Southern China. Hong Mai (the younger brother of Hong Zun) was a high-ranking civil official and had great interest in collecting occult anecdotes. His collection ended up in *Record of the Listener*, a series of books containing some 3,000 supernatural stories. Hong asserted that his stories were not fabricated and that the events described did take place; in his words, "All of the stories have their factual sources."[8] At the end of each, he often documented the informant's name and sometimes their occupation and social relations. Many informants claimed to have witnessed the anomalous events. By including such details, Hong enhanced the claimed historical factuality of his stories.

THE SONG PHYSICIANS' VIEW

The Song medical authors discussed in the four main chapters of this book were all scholar-officials who had either earned examination degrees or were civil officials. How did Song physicians consider and apply the empirical strategy? In general, when using persuasion strategies, they, even in the Southern Song period, preferred to demonstrate their command of various and numerous texts. Those they cited went beyond medical literature, extending to various literary and historical genres, such as poems, notebooks, and standard histories.

One case in point is Chen Yan, a physician who once lived in Yichun (in Jiangxi) and Yongjia (in Zhejiang) and wrote a pharmacological encyclopedia between 1227 and 1248. In the work, *Synthesizing Views on Materia Medica in the Baoqing Regime* (Baoqing bencao zhezhong), Chen cited a wide range of medical, literary, and historical genres. In addition to including numerous bookish references, he expressed a conservative view of the evidential value of witnesses. Chen claimed that he "witnessed" (*muji*) a great number of medicinal substances that originated near where he lived that had demonstrated therapeutic efficacy; however, "without seeing ancient people's evidence, I dared not arrogate to myself establishing entries [on those substances in my *Synthesizing Views on Materia Medica*]."[9] The evidence, on my reading, refers to earlier authors' writings about the therapeutic efficacy of those substances. Chen's words clearly prioritized authority derived from ancient texts over knowledge claims based on his empirical observation.[10]

Another instance of Song physicians' preferred persuasion strategies can be found in Yang Shiying's writings. As a physician who was active in Sanshan (in Fujian), Yang wrote four lengthy medical treatises and printed them in the 1260s. In them, he cited a wide spectrum of texts, ranging from medical works to Buddhist classics to notebooks (such as *Record of the Listener*).[11] When expressing his opinions, he wrote frequently as if they were matters of fact and rarely documented his successful practices to buttress the credibility of those opinions.

To be sure, some Song physicians recorded their healing practices in medical treatises that they wrote and published; however, those records occupy no central place in their works. This tendency is evident in *The Formulary for Saving Lives with Factual Evidence* (Huoren shizheng fang, hereafter *Formulary with Factual Evidence*) by Liu Xinfu (fl. early 13th century) and *Correcting Errors in the Easy and Concise Formulary* (Yijian fang jiumiu, hereafter *Correcting Errors*) by Lu Tan (fl. 13th century). Liu, like Xu Shuwei, had attended civil service examinations over many years, but was not as lucky as Xu. Facing ever-worsening odds against examination success in the thirteenth century, Liu never passed the examinations and eventually earned his living as a physician. He composed *The Formulary with Factual Evidence* in 1216, a title that reminds us of Zhu Gong's *Saving Lives* and Xu's *Formulary with Explanatory Historical Contexts*. In many formulas, Liu added case narratives that described successful cures and indicated witnesses' names. He described others' successful cures using almost the same format in which he narrated his own. The first-person pronoun used in some of the case narratives was often the only hint that an account of a successful outcome might have derived from Liu's own practice.

The similarity between the narrative formats in which Liu recorded his successful cures and others' cures suggests that his primary purpose in documenting case narratives was unlikely to have been stressing his own healing virtuosity. Instead, as shown in the phrase "factual evidence" in the formulary title, his purpose was more likely to provide testimony to the historical factuality of the efficacy of the remedies he recorded. This purpose closely resembled Shen Kuo's, Kou Zongshi's, Li Qiu's, and Wang Fei's purposes in documenting case narratives in their medical treatises. Liu's formulary enjoyed such wide popularity that he was asked, presumably by a commercial publisher, to write a sequel.[12] The subsequent work similarly includes the phrase "factual evidence" in its title.

Like Liu Xinfu, Lu Tan in his *Correcting Errors* did not push his case narratives into the foreground but devoted much more space to his diagnosis and prescription theories. Lu was a physician who was active in Yongjia, a prosperous region featuring a competitive medical marketplace. In *Correcting Errors*, he harshly criticized physicians and formularies that were popular there, such as that of his rival healer, Sun Zhining, as well as Sun's formulary. When disputing Sun's prescriptions in his formulary, Lu heavily relied on theoretical reasoning

CONCLUSION *137*

regarding diagnosis and pharmacological knowledge, such as correspondences between sets of symptoms and the effects and perceived natures of drugs. Another persuasion strategy Lu frequently deployed was citing medical classics and then elaborating on his interpretation of those quotations. The main texts that he quoted were *The Inner Canon* and *Treatise on Cold Damage*. Lu depicted Sun as a physician who not only misread the latter but also had little pharmacological knowledge.[13] Occasionally, Lu included case narratives, which served to illustrate his medical arguments and his interpretations of doctrinal texts.

Why did Song physicians, when applying persuasion strategies, tend to prioritize their erudition over presenting narratives of their successful cures? Before attempting to answer this question, we need to account for historiographic bias; that is, that the extant works of the Song physicians were, for the most part, composed by learned physicians, many of whom had prepared for and attended civil service examinations over the decades, becoming adept at composition. The less-educated healers—such as midwives, spirit mediums, and pharmacists—were by and large not literate enough to compose medical treatises or even to leave *any* words to us in our time, even though they outnumbered the learned physicians in the medical marketplace. This historiographic disproportion between the extant works of learned physicians and the work of less educated healers heavily conditions our understanding of the Song physicians' preferred persuasion strategies. When modern scholars discuss how various healing practitioners in the Song era built up their reputations via documentary media, the extant sources allow us to observe only how learned physicians promoted themselves.

Despite this bias, a significant portion of the explanation of the learned physicians' preference for the bookish strategy lies in the particular configuration of the medical marketplace in Song China. Competition already existed in earlier periods, but the establishment of the Imperial Pharmacy in the Song era greatly intensified that competition. The Song court established the pharmacy in the capital in 1076. It sold ready-made medicines to the public below market prices. In the late eleventh century, the court compiled *The Imperial Pharmacy's Formulary* (Taiyi ju fang).[14] This served as a self-help manual to help the sick and their caregivers choose and purchase formulas for medicines that were sold in the pharmacy. It thereby relieved individuals of the financial burden involved in consulting physicians. The Northern Song state fell shortly afterward.

In 1151, the Southern Song court reestablished the Imperial Pharmacy, editing and disseminating a new edition of *The Imperial Pharmacy's Formulary*, titled

138 CONCLUSION

The Formulary of the Bureau for Benefiting People and Compounding Formulations in an Era of Great Peace (Taiping huimin heji jufang). Several local governments then established branches of the pharmacy in their administrative prefectures, some of which were located in present-day Guangdong, Fujian, and Zhejiang. *The Imperial Pharmacy's Formulary* then underwent revision and expansion during the course of the Southern Song era and was printed at least twice in the Shaoxing regime (1131–1163) and again in 1208. The wider geographical distribution of the pharmacy and the printing of *The Imperial Pharmacy's Formulary* in the Southern Song era together provided the public with additional opportunities to choose cheaper, ready-made medicines than in the Northern Song period, which intensified competition in the medical marketplace. The formulary moreover empowered less-educated healers to ignore patients' individual bodily particularities by prescribing the pharmacy's ready-made medicines.[15] Learned physicians, in turn, stressed their erudition to defend their expertise and differentiate themselves from their less-educated competitors.

MEDICAL CASE NARRATIVES
IN PREMODERN CHINA AND EUROPE

The world in which Chinese physicians plied their trade had changed dramatically by the time the Ming state was founded in the fifteenth century. The Ming court retreated from active medical governance, ceasing to manage imperial pharmacies. Meanwhile, a printing boom expanded access to medical texts and accelerated the influx into the medical marketplace of both educated elites and others from lower social strata.[16] Facing the increasingly diverse marketplace, learned physicians in Ming China, unlike their Song counterparts, exhibited a more assertive attitude toward publishing collections of their case narratives as a means of self-promotion. Starting in the sixteenth century, ever-growing numbers of physicians began including their case narratives in their medical treatises, which they then printed. These narratives thus formed the bulk of these works' major content.

A shift in the role of case narratives occurred in the sixteenth century. A group of authors began to prioritize them over remedies in their treatises. Such treatises mark the emergence of a new genre of Chinese medical literature, which modern scholars have called the *yi'an* (medical case statements) genre. *Yi'an* authors were predominantly physicians and their disciples. In disseminating their books, they in general sought to recruit more disciples and to elevate the prestige of their own prescription styles and learning lineages.[17] While sharing a common aspiration, the Ming-era *yi'an* books exhibited variations in the literary styles through which cases were narrated and classified.[18] Bearing this variety in mind, we can gain further insight into changes and continuities of empirical evidence in medicine in imperial China through a comparison between the Song medical case narratives and those found in Ming-dynasty *yi'an* books.[19]

One obvious similarity between the Song case narratives and the Ming *yi'an* genre is their evidential function: both the Song and Ming case narratives in a given medical treatise served to buttress their reliability for publication. The chief aim of the majority of Song case narratives was to prove the historical factuality of the efficacy of recorded remedies. Some authors in the Song era attested to the attention given to factuality by including phrases such as "explanatory historical contexts" and "factual evidence" in their formulary titles. Although the narratives in the Ming *yi'an* genre still served this purpose, they additionally become significant and commonly used means of propagating a physician's expertise in diagnosis and prescription. Another, more important, similarity lies in their close association with pharmacology, especially with individually tailored prescriptions. Song and Ming medical authors often used their case narratives to emphasize the importance of tailoring pharmacological knowledge to each sick person's symptomatic and bodily particularities (one thinks here, for example, of the five difficulties Shen Kuo discussed). In the Song era, this emphasis often appeared as a concern about standardized remedies that the government enthusiastically provided to treat the public and to teach and transform laypersons. In the Ming era, during which government medical activism diminished considerably, the emphasis appeared more often in the context of debates between rival healers regarding diagnosis and treatment as they vied to win patients' patronage.

Song medical case narratives differed from those in the Ming *yi'an* genre in three major respects: the scope over which cases were collected, the degree to which authors were aware of the narrative as a form of medical writing, and fields of knowledge related to medical cases. The most apparent difference is in the scope of a collection. Extant Song sources leave us no clues regarding the existence of collections in which the cases were taken from a single person's healing practice. In Song treatises in which case narratives form the major part (such as Xu Shuwei's *Formulary with Explanatory Historical Contexts* and Liu Xinfu's *Formulary with Factual Evidence*), those records always came from multiple healing practitioners, who often lived centuries apart and so no master-disciple relationships were involved. For their part, many Ming authors compiled anthologies of case narratives. One example is *Classified Cases from Famous Physicians* (Mingyi leian, completed in 1552, but printed in 1591). Beginning in the sixteenth century, however, late imperial–period case collections representing individual practitioners appeared with increasing frequency. Three early instances are *Sayings of a Female Doctor*, *Stone Mountain Medical Cases*, and *Mr. Han's Generalities on Medicine* (Hanshi yitong, 1522).

The abovementioned differences in the scope of the collected cases relates to vital elements that established the credibility of case narratives. The credibility of a Song case narrative was built primarily on the specificity of the information it conveyed, which could include the authors' witnesses, names, occupations, the social relations of persons who attended the event, informants' names and backgrounds, and geographical locations and times of day. With few exceptions, in the Song period, an author's expertise in medicine was not the central element establishing the credibility of a case narrative, whereas in the Ming *yi'an* genre, the central element became the main actor's medical expertise.[20]

In comparison with Song medical authors, Ming authors working in the *yi'an* genre demonstrated much greater awareness of the case narrative as a form of medical writing. This heightened awareness is evident in the Ming authors' efforts to design a structured format for recording them. For instance, Han Mao in his *Mr. Han's Generalities on Medicine* proposed a format that began with "in place X [relating to] person Y on date Z, I fill out this medical case" and then described in sequence the patient's figure, height, appearance (such as being "glossy" [*run*] or "withered" [*gao*]), sound, pitch, pulse patterns, and so forth.[21] In a similar vein, Wu Kun in his *Language of Pulse Patterns* (Maiyu) proposed another structured format.[22] As Han Mao envisioned it, a case record following his format could not only prevent a physician from omitting important points in making a diagnosis but also could help a patient save the record and then consult other physicians for their opinions.[23] Ming authors never quite made case records in structured formats prevalent, and even Wu and Han in their writings did not strictly follow the format they proposed. Nevertheless, the Ming authors' proposed structured format testifies to their awareness of the case narrative as a particular medium for transmitting medical knowledge and physicians' professional capacity.

Song medical authors, in contrast, demonstrated little interest in forming a

CONCLUSION   *141*

structured sequence of steps when narrating a case, and provided no guidelines for writing them up. Although they wrote without following a structured format, Song authors by no means documented what happened as free-form notations. They seemed to share a tacit understanding that a case narrative at least included informants' information, such as their names or social backgrounds.

When explaining why they recorded case narratives in writing, Song medical authors analogized physicians' decision-making to decisions made on battlefields. For instance, Wei Xian in *Mr. Wei's Family Collection of Formulas* cited the words of the famous Northern Song scholar Shao Yong (1012–1077), who observed that "applying drugs to attack disorders is like joining soldiers in battle."[24] Another example comes from the preface to *The Formulary with Factual Evidence*. The author of the preface, Ye Linzhi, argued that "physicians attacking disorders is like 'military strategists' (*bingjia*) attacking enemies." He praised the case narratives collected in this formulary for enabling readers to make informed decisions about treatments. Ye considered this pedagogic usefulness similar to that of military books for military strategists.[25] The analogy between physicians and military strategists was still commonplace in late imperial writings.

When explaining the usefulness of *yi'an* books, Ming authors frequently appealed to perceived similarities between medical cases and legal cases.[26] These similarities, however, rarely appeared in Song authors' explanations. For instance, Cheng Lu, the author of the preface to *Stone Mountain Medical Cases*, believed that one benefit of this treatise was that "when those who came after peruse the case narrative, isn't it just like the use made by legal experts of settled cases?"[27] The accumulation of medical case narratives, like that of legal cases, was thought to serve potentially as a historical archive to help succeeding learners make pertinent medical decisions. After *Stone Mountain Medical Cases*, *yi'an* literature often drew parallels between physicians' decision-making in clinical situations and that of legal officials' in the judicial process. Wu Kun appealed to this parallel as follows: "When medicines get to work and the disorders in question hide away, one must act like an experienced legal official hearing a case, who cites the law and fixes the penalty so that the guilty have no place to go."[28] Modern scholarship has pointed out that the Ming authors' likening of medical cases to legal ones involved analogizing diagnosis to interrogating a subject, analogizing efforts to discern the etiologies of disorders to obtaining a confession, and analogizing prescribing medicines to citing laws and rendering a verdict.[29]

142 CONCLUSION

Comparison of Song medical case narratives with those found in Ming *yi'an* literature reveals important variations over time. Some features of the former are reminiscent of findings in scholarship on the development of the case narrative in medical genres in Europe.[30] To be very brief, in premodern Europe, physicians consistently recorded their own successful cures. In the middle decades of the sixteenth century, however, they began publishing collections of those records, which they called *curationes, observationes*, and *historiae*. These were published primarily to tout a physician's expertise and fame. Before that, published case narratives were inserted as anecdotes or examples in medical texts. Although there existed a genre devoted to cases, the *consilium*, its aim was to define them within the framework of doctrinal knowledge. Song medical authors likewise often appended a case narrative before or after describing a remedy (usually a drug formula) and sometimes used the narrative to illustrate a theoretical argument that they drew or developed from medical classics.

On the one hand, case narratives developed similarly in China and Europe before the sixteenth century: in both cases, they functioned merely as textual examples but did not acquire a distinctive status in medical writings. On the other hand, the medical learning environments in medieval Europe and Song China were very different. In Europe, case narratives were transmitted mainly as private records in manuscripts that were passed from masters to disciples or within a teacher's *familia*. In China, although medical knowledge was often transmitted within a family and through an apprenticeship, autodidacts who acquired it through reading were plentiful. To persuade such self-taught practitioners, Song authors highlighted their own case narratives (and other accounts based on personal experience) as evidence of the reliability of their writings. The evidential power of these comes not from interpersonal familiarity between authors and readers but rather from the historical factuality that authors claimed for it.[31]

Empiricism as a mode of verifying therapeutic efficacy continued to underpin medical authority in both Europe and China in the centuries that followed the historical eras on which this book has focused. Hands-on testing of drugs was central to medicine and the rise of scientific experiments in early modern Europe.[32] In early twentieth-century China, when not only Western biomedicine but also the Chinese government seriously questioned the legitimacy of classical Chinese medicine, its advocates launched a number of measures to reinstate their authority.[33] One such measure involved highlighting the empirical tradition, characterizing classical Chinese medicine as an experience (*jingyan*)-centered healing praxis. Those advocates set up a relationship of opposition between classical Chinese medicine and Western biomedicine by declaring that the former was based on "experience with the human body" whereas the latter relied on "animal experiments." Chinese medicine, they claimed, was accordingly more appropriate for application to human bodies. This opposition was not merely a rhetorical strategy, as it affected the protocol for scientific research on Chinese drugs in modern China.[34] Even in our own time, supporters of traditional Chinese medicine (TCM) still hotly debate the relative benefits of pragmatic and clinical trials as standards of scientific proof in TCM. In this sense, how to prove therapeutic efficacy to the public continues to haunt TCM communities today as much as it troubled Song-dynasty men of letters.

Song authors' efforts to establish the reliability of knowledge to be published (via manuscripts or stone inscriptions, or in print) occurred not only in medical literature but also in many literary and historical writings during this period. The life-and-death nature of healing knowledge, however, gives such efforts extra weight when medical knowledge was involved. The challenge involved in ensuring a published treatise's reliability had ancient roots: the absence of any threshold for writing and publishing medical texts since the classical age in China, when any literate and resourceful author could compile, compose, and circulate such treatises. In addition to these ancient roots, the challenge intensified following the boom in medical text publishing in the Song era, when authors endeavored to prove the credibility and trustworthiness of the treatises they wrote and published, employing several persuasion strategies. Among these, highlighting the evidential value of the empirical strategy was often chosen. The authors' efforts to make knowledge trustworthy during the publishing boom, with no threshold of truth over which they had to pass, even across a span of eight hundred years, echoes our contemporary struggle to build a system that ensures the reliability of knowledge claims in the face of an information explosion.

Glossary of Chinese Characters

NOTE: Chinese characters for authors and book titles cited in the notes can be found in the bibliography.

ai 艾
Ai Sheng 艾晟

Bai Juyi 白居易
Baihu Tang 白虎湯
Bao Tingbo 鮑廷博
beihu 北戶
beiyi 北醫
bencao 本草
Bencao gangmu shiyi 本草綱目拾遺
Bencao tujing 本草圖經
benshi 本事
Benshifang houji 本事方後集
bi 閉
Bian shanghan 辨傷寒
bianji 辨疾
bianjiao Zhaowen Guan shuji
　編校昭文館書籍
Bianlei 辨類
bianyao 辨藥
bieben 別本
Bieci shanghan 別次傷寒
biejia 鱉甲
bieyao 別藥

biji 筆記
bing 病
bingan 病案
bingjia 兵家
bo 博
bowu 博物
Buhuan Jin Zhengqi San 不換金正氣散

cai 採
cao gu shu 草蠱術
Cao Xiaozhong 曹孝忠
caozi 草子
chaihu 柴胡
chen 沉
Chen Baxian 陳霸先
Chen Cangqi 陳藏器
Chen Cheng 陳承
Chen Yaosou 陳堯叟
Cheng Yongpei 程永培
chi 尺
chong 蟲
*Chongguang buzhu Shennong bencao bing
　tujing* 重廣補注神農本草並圖經
Chuanxin fang 傳信方

chufang 處方
Chunyu Yi 淳于意
ci 賜
cihua 詞話
Cui Zhiti 崔知悌
Cuishi zuanyaogfang 崔氏纂要方

Da Chaihu Tang 大柴胡湯
dahuang 大黃
daimao 玳瑁
daizhi 待制
danggui 當歸
dangshi shishi 當時事實
dao 道
Daozang jing 道藏經
Datang xiyuji 大唐西域記
Didang Tang 抵當湯
dong bitu 東壁土
du 度 (degrees)
du 毒 (poison/potency)
Du Fu 杜甫
Du Mu 杜牧

Erya 爾雅

fabiao 發表
fan 煩
Fan Yun 范雲
Fang Qianli 房千里
fangji 方技
fangshu 方書
fangzhong 房中
fengdu 風毒
fu 浮
Furen daquan liangfang 婦人大全良方
fuyu 俘鬱

gan 感
gao 槁

Gao Baoheng 高保衡
Gao Roune 高若訥
Gegen Tang 葛根湯
gewu 格物
gewu zhizhi 格物致知
gongshiku 公使庫
gu 蠱
guange 館閣
guange jiaokan
　　館閣校勘
Guangnan shesheng fang lun
　　廣南攝生方論
Guangnan sishi shesheng fang lun
　　廣南四時攝生方論
Guangnan sishi sheyang kuozi
　　廣南四時攝養括子
gui 桂
Guilin fengtu ji 桂林風土記
Gujin jiyanfang 古今集驗方
Guozi Jian 國子監
guyang jiao 羖羊角

han 汗
Han Qi 韓琦
Han Yu 韓愈
Hanlin xueshi 翰林學士
hanshan 寒疝
He Yujuan 何與狷
hedong 河東
Hongwen Guan 弘文館
hou 候
houxu 後序
Hu Mian 胡勉
Huang Tingjian 黃庭堅
Huangdi neijing 黃帝內經
Huangfu mi 皇甫謐
huangqi 黃芪
huo 或
Huoren zhinan 活人指南

huowen 或問

huoyue 或曰

Ishimpō 醫心方

ji 疾 (disorders)

ji 給 (provide)

ji 技 (techniques)

Jiahe San 嘉禾散

jiang 漿

jianwen 見聞

Jianzhong Tang 建中湯

jiaohua 教化

jiaoqi 腳氣

jiaoruo 腳弱

Jiaozheng Yishuju 校正醫書局

Jiaozhou yiwu zhi 交州異物志

Jiayi jing 甲乙經

Jiayou buzhu Shennong bencao
　嘉祐補註神農本草

jiexian 疥癬

jiguan 籍貫

jiji 几几

jijia 疾瘕

jin 斤

jing 經 (canons)

jing 經 (channels)

jingfang 經方

jingguan 京官

Jingling bayou 竟陵八友

Jingshi zhenglei beiji bencao
　經史證類備急本草

Jingshi zhenglei daguan bencao
　經史證類大觀本草

jingtian 景天

Jingxiao leili 經效類例

jingyan 經驗

jingyao 精要

jinshi 進士

jinye 津液

jiuben 舊本

Jixian Guan 集賢館

Jiyan fang 集驗方

juan 卷

jueli 厥理

Kaibao xinxiangding bencao
　開寶新詳定本草

ke 客

Kou Yue 寇約

Kou Zhun 寇準

Kuizhou tujing 夔州圖經

Laigong xunlie 萊公勳烈

laoyi 老醫

leishu 類書

Leizheng puji benshifang xuji
　類證普濟本事方續集

Li Bai 李白 (701–762)

Li Bo 李渤 (fl. early 9th century)

Li Daoyuan 酈道元

Li Qiu 李璆

Li Xuan 李暄

Li Zhuguo 李柱國

li 理 (coherence)

li 利 (disinhibit)

Liang Wudi 梁武帝

Liangfang 良方

liangyi 良醫

Liao shanghan shen yan fang
　療傷寒身驗方

Lin Yi 林億

Lingbiao shishuo 嶺表十說

Lingnan 嶺南

Lingnan fang 嶺南方

Lingnan jiaoqi lun 嶺南腳氣論

Lingnan jiyao fang 嶺南急要方

Lingshu 靈樞

Liu Ke 劉克
Liu Xun 劉恂
Lizhi pu 荔枝譜
Lu Xisheng 陸希聲
luci 鸕鷀
lun 論
luo 絡

Ma Yuan 馬援
mahuang 麻黃
maixi 脈息
man 漫
meiyao 媚藥
men 悶
mifeng cao 蜜蜂草
min 憫
Mingyi leian 名醫類案
minjian 民間
Mo Xiufu 莫休符
mudu 目睹
muji 目擊
mujian 目見
Muxiang Wan 木香丸

nan bitu 南壁土
nanren 南人
Nanzhou yiwuzhi 南州異物志
nüe 瘧
Nüyi zayan 女醫雜言

pi 痞
pingwei 平胃
Pingwei San 平胃散
poxiao 朴硝
pu 僕
pulu 譜錄

qi 其
Qibao Cuo San 七寶銼散

qieyi 竊意
qifang shanshu 奇方善術
qihai 氣海
Qilüe 七略
qing 情
qinghao 青蒿
qinjian 親見
qiong jiang 瓊漿
quzhe 曲折

ren 人
Ren Hong 任宏
rongqi 榮氣
ru 儒
ruchen 儒臣
run 潤
ruyi 儒醫
ruyong 乳癰

sanli 三里
Sanshiliu shuifa 三十六水法
se 澀
shafu 砂俘
shan zhangnüe 山瘴瘧
shanghan 傷寒
Shanghan fawei lun 傷寒發微論
Shanghan leili 傷寒類例
Shanghan maijue 傷寒脈訣
Shanghan zongbing lun 傷寒總病論
Shanghan zuanlei 傷寒纂類
Shangshu Sheng 尚書省
shanren 山人
shanyao 山藥
Shao Yong 邵雍
Shaoxing jiaoding bencao 紹興校定本草
Shen Pi 沈披
Shengjiang Fuzi Tang 生薑附子湯
Shennong bencao jing 神農本草經
shenxian 神仙

Shenyi pujiu fang 神醫普救方
Shesheng lun 攝生論
shi 實 (factual)
shi 勢 (propensity)
shi 士 (scholars, literati)
shi du qi 濕毒氣
Shi Guan 史館
shidafu 士大夫
Shijing 詩經
shiren 市人
shishi 實事
Shiwu jiyuan 事物紀原
Shixian benshi quziji 時賢本事曲子集
shiyi 侍醫
Shizhongshan ji 石鍾山記
shoujin 瘦金
Shoumai Yaocaisuo 收買藥材所
shu 暑
Shuijing zhu 水經注
shumi shi 樞密使
Su Mai 蘇邁
Suhexiang Wan 蘇合香丸
sui 隨
Sun Qi 孫奇
Sun Zhao 孫兆
Sun Zhining 孫志寧
Suwen 素問

Taisu 太素
taiyang 太陽
Taiyi ju fang 太醫局方
Taiyi Xue 太醫學
Tanba Yasuyori 丹波康賴
Tanluan 曇鸞
tianniu chong 天牛蟲
tiao 條
tiao caozi 挑草子
Tiaoqi fang 調氣方
tongxi 通犀

Tongzhen zi shanghan kuoyao
　通真子傷寒括要
Touhuang zalu 投荒雜錄

Wang Fangqing 王方慶
Wang Fei 王棐
Wang Nanrong 汪南容
Wang Shi 王寔
Wangshi boji fang 王氏博濟方
wei 味
wenji 文集
wenjian 聞見
wu 物 (objects/things)
wu 巫 (spirit mediums)
wugui 烏鬼
wuhuo 無惑
wunan 五難
Wuqiuzi shanghan baiwen
　無求子傷寒百問
wuxing 五行

xia 下
xian 弦
Xianjing 仙經
xianwei 縣尉
xiao 鴞
Xiao Chaihu Tang 小柴胡湯
Xiao Chengqi Tang 小承氣湯
Xiao Jianzhong Tang 小建中湯
Xiao Yan 蕭衍
Xiaoer yaozheng zhenjue 小兒藥證真訣
xiaoshuo 小說
xie 洩
Xie Fugu 謝復古
xin 信
Xinbian zhenglei tuzhu bencao
　新編證類圖註本草
xinfu zhangji 心腹脹急
xing 性

GLOSSARY OF CHINESE CHARACTERS　*149*

Xinxiu bencao 新修本草
xinyi 新意
xu 虛 (deficient)
xu 畜 (store)
Xu Xueshi 許學士
xuanren 選人
xue 血 (blood)
xue 學 (learning)
Xue Jinghui 薛景晦
xuezhe 學者
xuhan 虛寒
xuli 序例

yan 驗
Yan Shigu 顏師古
yanfang 驗方 (effective formulas)
yanfang 炎方 (terroir of flame)
Yang Hui 楊繪
Yang Shiying 楊士瀛
yangming 陽明
yanshu 鼴鼠
yaoshen 妖神
Yaoyi 藥議
yazhang 啞瘴
Ye Linzhi 葉麟之
yi 藝 (arts)
yi 醫 (medicine)
Yi shanghan lun 翼傷寒論
yi'an 醫案
yidao 醫道
yifang 醫方
yijing 醫經
yinyao 飲藥
yishi 醫士
yishu 醫書
yiwu zhi 異物志
Yixue 醫學
yixue boshi 醫學博士
yiyi shi 薏苡實

Yizhen zhi 儀真志
yu 鬱 (compressed)
yu 余 (I)
yu 愚 (I, in my state of ignorance)
Yu Yanguo Lixian Tang 余彥國勵賢堂
yubi 御筆
Yueling 月令
yujiang 玉漿
yun 云
yun qi 運氣
yuquan 玉泉
yushui 玉水
yuxue 瘀血
yuzhang 禦瘴

za 雜
zadu 雜毒
zhang 瘴 (miasma)
zhang 障 (obstacles)
Zhang Chan 張蕆
Zhang Jie 章杰
Zhang Yu 張遇
Zhang Zhiyuan 張致遠
zhangdu jiaoqi 瘴毒腳氣
zhangji 瘴疾
zhangli 瘴癘
Zhanglun 瘴論
Zhangnüe lun 瘴瘧論
zhangqi 瘴氣
zhangyi 瘴疫
Zhao Xuemin 趙學敏
Zhaowen Guan 昭文館
Zheng Jingxiu 鄭景岫
*Zhenghe xinxiu jingshi zhenglei beiyong
    bencao* 政和新修經史證類備用本草
zhengqi 正氣
zhenji 診籍
Zhifa bashiyi pian 治法八十一篇
zhiji 治疾

Zhimi fang zhang nüe lun
指迷方瘴瘧論

Zhongjing maifa sanshiliu tu
仲景脈法三十六圖

zhongwan 中脘

zhongzhou 中州

Zhouhou jiuzu 肘後救卒

zhubu 主簿

zhuzhi 主治

zi 自 (grounds)

zi 字 (style names)

zonghao 總號

zongzu 宗族

Notes

Introduction

1. Scholars have rendered Shen's given name alternately as "Kuo" and "Gua" ("Kua" was used in Wade-Giles romanization, which has been replaced by the People's Republic of China's pinyin system).

2. *Su Shen neihan liangfang*, 5.714. The basic format of medical formulas in imperial China is a list of disorders it could treat and of ingredients followed by detailed instructions for preparing the ingredients and administering remedies.

3. For further comparison between the Western notion of experience and the Chinese concept of *jingyan* (experience) in philosophical terms, see Zuo, *Shen Gua's Empiricism*, 14–18.

4. Shapin and Schaffer, *Leviathan*, 25–26. Their book has challenged the conventional understanding of the Scientific Revolution by showing that scientific knowledge claims were not internally produced by an esoteric scientific community but instead shaped by social dynamics involving a wide range of actors who operated outside of it.

5. Patricia Ebrey and Peter Bol used the term "middle period China" in 2014 at the Conference on Middle Period China, 800–1400. The term provides a time frame that is broader than a dynasty, is "less Eurocentric than 'medieval,' and does not carry associations of decline from a classical era." Ebrey and Huang, *Visual and Material Cultures*, 1.

6. Hinrichs, "Governance through Medical Texts"; and *Shamans, Witchcraft, and Quarantine*. I am immensely grateful to Prof. Hinrichs for sharing her manuscript with me.

7. For more on the contrasts between printing cultures in early modern China and Europe, see Brokaw, "On the History of the Book."

8. For recent studies on the impacts of printing technology in middle-period China, see Chia and De Weerdt, eds., *Knowledge and Text Production*.

9. Fried, "Song Dynasty Classicism."

10. On recent statistics of medical imprints in the Song, see Chen Ruth Yun-ju, "Songdai shidafu canyu difang yishu kanyin xintan."

11. Cherniack, "Book Culture"; Wang Yugen, *Ten Thousand Scrolls*. Other significant studies on this transformation that informed this book are cited in later chapters.

12. McDermott, *Social History*, 43–82.

13. On the importance of being initiated by a master into the art of healing in early China, see Sivin, "Text and Experience," 177–88; and Li Jianmin, "Zhongguo gudai jinfang kaolun."

14. Harper, *Early Chinese Medical Literature*, 55–67; Chin, *Zhongguo gudai de yixue, yishi, yu zhengzhi*, 86–98, and "Chutu gudai yiliao xiangguan wenben de shuxie yu bianci"; Brown, *Art of Medicine*.

15. Fan, "Weijinnanbeichao Sui Tang shiqi de yixue," 162–69; Chen Hao, *Shenfen xushi yu zhishi biaoshu zhijian de yizhe zhiyi*, 87–161; Dolly Yang, "Prescribing 'Guiding and Pulling.'"

16. On Tang officials' practice of collecting and circulating medical formulas, see Fan, *Zhonggu shiqi de yizhe yu bingzhe*, 153–85.

17. For the formulation see, Goldschmidt, *Evolution of Chinese Medicine*, 199. For English-language scholarship adopting this formulation, for instance, see, Sivin, *Health Care*.

18. Sivin, "Text and Experience," 190–95.

19. The shift in the criteria that qualify empirical evidence as reliable discussed in this book helps reveal changes in, as some historians put it, "cultures of reasoning" in imperial China. Cultures of reasoning exist through "inter-subjectively accepted mechanisms for claiming and assessing the validity of textual evidence, empirical observations, and argumentative strategies." For studies of cultures of reasoning in imperial China, but with a focus on the seventeenth and nineteenth centuries, see Hofmann, Kurtz, and Levine, eds., *Powerful Arguments*.

20. Medical case narratives in imperial China generally included basic information about the sick (such as social position, gender, age, disease history, and name), diagnoses, and treatments.

21. Studies of "medical case statements" in imperial China have analyzed their epistemic function, the socio-intellectual contexts surrounding their emergence and popularity, and the healing practices they reveal. The studies are too numerous to cite exhaustively here. For seminal studies that investigate the popularity of this new genre against the prevailing "style of thinking" in late imperial China, see Furth, Zeitlin, and Hsiung, eds., *Thinking with Cases*. Recent studies, such as Marta Hanson's *Speaking of Epidemics in Chinese Medicine*, examine the practice of documenting authors' personal experience in other medical literature of late imperial China.

22. Sima, *Shiji*, 105.3381, 3400.

23. For a careful analysis of medical cases in Chunyu Yi's biography and the bodily experience involved in such cases, see Hsu, *Pulse Diagnosis*. Scholarly opinions have been divided on the authorship of the twenty-five medical cases. For a recent review of these opinions, see Brown, *Art of Medicine*, 77–86.

24. Furth, "Producing Medical Knowledge," 131–51; Cullen, "*Yi'an* (Case Statements)," 309–21.

25. Andrews, "From Case Records." On the competition between Chinese medicine and Western medicine during this period, see, for instance, Lei, *Neither Donkey nor Horse*.

26. Hanson and Pomata, "Medicinal Formulas."

27. On the birth and development of *observationes*, see Pomata, "Sharing Cases."

28. Pomata, "Medical Case Narrative."

29. One exception is He Bian's recent article, which suggests that physicians and elite patients were both invested in the production of medical cases. See Bian, "Documenting Medications."

30. Furth, "Producing Medical Knowledge," 126–31; Cullen, "*Yi'an* (Case Statements)," 309. One exception that challenges this view is *Ninety Discussions on Cold Damage Disorders* (Shanghan jiushi lun), a single-author medical case collection attributed to a Song author. Whether *Ninety Discussions* was a Song-dynasty work is still, however, open to scholarly dispute. In chapter 3, I discuss this dispute and explain why *Ninety Discussions* was in all likelihood *not* completed during the Song. On the translation and analysis of *Ninety Discussions*, see Goldschmidt, *Medical Practice*.

31. Burke, *What Is the History*.

32. For recent English-language studies on the popularity of composing notebooks, travel literature, and inventories of things in the Song era, see, De Pee, "Notebooks (*biji*) and Shifting Boundaries"; Hargett, *Jade Mountains*, 90–121; Mai, "Double Life"; and Siebert, "Consuming and Possessing Things" and "Animal as Text."

33. On the expanding scope of civil service examinations in the Song era, see Chaffee, *Thorny Gates of Learning*.

34. Studies of the Tang-Song transition of ruling elites originated in what scholars call the "Naitō hypothesis." Naitō Torajirō (1866–1934) proposed this hypothesis, provoking a large body of English-language, Japanese, and Chinese-language studies that examine and expand on it. For a summary of the hypothesis, see Miyakawa, "Outline of the Naitō Hypothesis."

35. For classic studies on the shift in the definition of cultural elites in the Song era, see Hymes, *Statesmen and Gentlemen*; Bol, *This Culture of Ours*; and Bossler, *Powerful Relations*.

36. On Song notebooks as examples of an informal prose style, see Hargett, "Sketches."

NOTES TO PAGES 6–9   155

37. On the difficulties involved in defining *biji*, see Bol, "Literati Miscellany," 124–27. For modern scholars' definitions of notebooks, see, among others, Liu Yeqiu, *Lidai biji gaishu*, 5; and Fu, "Flourishing of *Biji*."

38. On the 155 figures, see Zhang Hui, *Songdai biji yanjiu*, 31. On the 1,103 figures, see Gu, *Liang Song biji yanjiu*, 12–15.

39. Ellen Cong Zhang, "To Be 'Erudite in Miscellaneous Knowledge.'"

40. De Weerdt, *Information, Territory, and Networks*, 285–86.

41. For a study on the application of these methods in the Song era, see, among others, Inglis, *Hong Mai's Record*. For oral anecdotes as an important information source for notebook authors in the same period, see Ellen Cong Zhang, "Of Revelers"; and Hymes, "Gossip as History."

42. Zuo, *Shen Gua's Empiricism*, 172.

43. Inglis, *Hong Mai's Record*, 123–25; Zuo, *Shen Gua's Empiricism*, 175–85, 228–35.

44. Ban, *Han shu*, 30.1776–80.

45. As noted by many historians of Chinese medicine, the term *yi* in ancient and imperial China covers a much wider spectrum of concepts and practices than modern biomedicine does, as the former pertains both to healing practices and techniques for promoting vitality and achieving longevity. On the rich array of such practices and techniques, see Hinrichs and Barnes, eds., *Chinese Medicine and Healing*.

46. A similar methodology is adopted in the study of empiricism in early modern Europe. See Crisciani, "Histories, Stories, Exempla, and Anecdotes," 298.

47. Zuo, *Shen Gua's Empiricism*, 17–18. While both Zuo's monograph and this book address empiricism in the Song era, the research for the two studies was carried out in distinct time periods and applies distinct approaches to this topic. Zuo's monograph discusses features of empiricism in the context of learning between the eleventh and thirteenth centuries, covering the intellectual history of empiricism in Song China. This book explores specific historical contexts from which the empirical strategy arose and traces this strategy back to the ninth century, revealing the social and cultural history of empiricism in late Tang and Song China.

ONE New Criteria for "Good" Medical Formulas

1. Lo, "Han Period," 40.

2. In comparison, in her study of Middle English medical formulas, Claire Jones identified a group of Latin phrases that were appended at the ends of those formulas to promote their effects. She argued that those Latin phrases served to indicate that the formulas originated in ancient theoretical texts rather than providing empirical proof. See Jones, "Formula and Formulation."

3. Apart from building credibility, another relevant interpretation of the significance

of accompanying a formula with its applicants' official positions and surnames views the inclusion of such information as a selling point. Brown used the latter interpretation in her analysis of a medical formula that contains the phrase "a formula of General Geng of Jianwei" in its main text. The formula is dated to the first century CE and was discovered on the Wuwei frontier (in Gansu) in 1972. See Brown, *Art of Medicine*, 84.

4. For Sun Simiao's innovation in the production of medical knowledge and the analysis of the twenty-five cases, see Yan Liu, *Healing with Poisons*, 105–24. For a translation and brief discussion of some of the twenty-five cases, see Sivin, "Seventh-Century."

5. For Cui Zhiti's medical learning, see Chen Hao, *Ji zhi cheng shang*, 256–62.

6. *Waitai miyao fang*, 3.44.

7. *Waitai miyao fang*, 33.662–63. For an investigation into *Mr. Cui*'s author and an analysis of Tanluan's story about assisting with a newborn delivery, see Lee Jen-der, "Han Tang zhijian yishu zhongde shengchan zhi dao." For the English translation of this story, see Lee Jen-der, "Gender and Medicine in Tang China."

8. On the case histories in *Mr. Cui* and *Essential Formulas* and on the intellectual contexts in which those case histories emerged, see Chen Hao, *Shenfen xushi yu zhishi biaoshu zhijiande yizhe zhi yi*, 177–82. In that book Chen also proposes that, in the Tang dynasty, the practice of narrating a healing event using a first-person pronoun appears in scholar-officials' formularies more frequently than in others' formularies. Nevertheless, considering the paucity of Tang formularies that have come down to us, it is difficult in my view for historians to confirm that phenomenon.

9. Wang Tao, of the Institute for Extending Literature (Hongwen Guan), taking advantage of his access as an official to the imperial library, collected a considerable number of medical formulas from the library and brought them together to create *The Imperial Library Formulary* in 752.

10. Tamba Yasuyori, a physician in the Japanese court in the Heian period (ca. 794–1194), selected and transcribed Chinese medical writings up to the Tang era and then compiled them into *Formulas at the Heart of Medicine*. Two hundred and four Chinese medical works are cited in it, according to Ma Jixing, *Zhongyi wenxian xue*, 207.

11. Genette, *Paratexts*, 79–89.

12. Hanson, "From under the Elbow." Hanson uses the thematic/rhematic method to demonstrate how metaphors in book titles served to convey the contents, material forms, and textual innovations of medical "handbooks" in middle-period China. Indebted to her research, I use the method to disclose how authors featured reliability and empirical evidence in book titles from the same period.

13. Wei, *Sui shu*, 34.1042.

14. *Liu Yuxi quanji biannian jiaozhu*, 1037–38. Fan examined sources of information about the formulas in *Passing on Trustworthy Formulas* in the context of Tang officials'

emphasis on the value of formulas that were known to be effective. Fan, *Dayi jingcheng*, 147–68. Received parts of Liu's formulary are collected and edited in Feng Hanyong, *Gu fangshu jiyi*, 105–20.

15. *Boji fang*, 1.

16. *Shen Kuo quanji*, 28.178. My translation is based on Zuo, *Shen Gua's Empiricism*, 198.

17. For example, Sivin, based on this quotation, argued that "Shen's most characteristic contribution was undoubtedly his emphasis on his own experience." Sivin, "Shen Kua," 30. For a recent review of a considerable number of studies on Shen Kuo and his oeuvre, see Zuo, *Shen Gua's Empiricism*, 8–27.

18. *Shen Kuo quanji*, 28.177–78.

19. *Shen Kuo quanji*, 28.178. My translation is based on Boyanton, *"Treatise on Cold Damage,"* 76.

20. One revealing contrast with Shen Kuo's silence is that, sometime between 1227 and 1248, the Song physician Chen Yan, when writing down his reflections on Shen's preface, used "ways of medicine" (*yidao*) to refer to the ineffable profoundness that Shen evokes. *Baoqing bencao zhezhong,* 2.458.

21. *Sima Guang ji*, 27.678.

22. *Shen Kuo quanji*, 28.178.

23. *Shen Kuo quanji*, 28.178–79.

24. Fan, "*Ge Xianweng zhouhou beijifang*"; Stanley-Baker, "JY146 *Ge Xianweng zhouhou beiji fang.*"

25. The printed version bears the title *Newly Carved Immortal Sun's Formulary Worth a Thousand in Gold* (Xindiao Sun zhenren qianjin fang). For an investigation into the printing date and publishers of this version, see Zeng, "*Xindiao Sun zhenren qianjin fang* kanke niandai kao" and "*Xindiao Sun zhenren qianjin fang* kezhe kao."

26. On the circulation of *Essential Formulas* as hand-copied manuscripts and printed texts in the Song era, see Chen Hao, "Zai xieben yu yinben zhijian de fangshu."

27. A similar expression of the concept that no formula had universal effects appears in a later Song-era formulary, *Shi Zaizhi's Formulary* (Shi Zaizhi fang). Its author, Shi Kan (fl. 1086–1102), was famous for his medical expertise and obtained the advanced-scholar degree sometime between 1111 and 1118. In a section on diarrhea, Shi argues that physicians should modify treatments in accordance with specific subtypes of diarrhea, declaring that "this is why I think what formularies recorded were not formulas of inevitable effects." *Shi Zaizhi fang, xia*, 93.

28. *Beiji qianjin yaofang*, 1.1–13.

29. For a close analysis of *Su's and Shen's Formulas*, see Yi, "Songdai de shiren yu yifang."

30. *Junzhai dushuzhi jiaozheng*, 15.730.

31. For a survey of the editions and circulation of *Good Formulas* and *Su's and Shen's Formulas*, see Hu, "*Su Shen neihan liangfang* Chu Shu pan," 196–97; *Zhizhai shulu jieti*, 13.388; and *Suichutang shumu*, 494.

32. Hu, "*Su Shen neihan liangfang* chu shu pan," 87–112. The total of 252 items is based on the item numbers that Hu Daojing gave to each of the entries in *Su's and Shen's Formulas*. The figure 172 indicating how many items Shen Kuo wrote is based on existing studies and my analysis of *Su's and Shen's Formulas*. Hu identified 172 items that Shen wrote. Li Shuhui showed that items no. 132 and no. 225, the author of which Hu did not identify, were written by Shen. Li argued meanwhile that it was Su Shi who composed items no. 49 and no. 179a, two that Hu identified as Shen's. Because Li did not give concrete evidence of Su Shi as the author of item no. 49, however, I regard its authorship as unknown. See Li Shuhui, "*Su Shen liangfang* zuozhe qufen xinkao" and "*Su Shen liangfang* zuozhe qufen xinkao (xuwan)."

33. Yi Sumei noticed the contrast as well but did not explain why it occurred. Yi, "Songdai de shiren yu yifang," 89.

34. Hu, "*Su Shen neihan liangfang* Chu Shu pan," 197–99. Items 039, 058B, 063, 086, 090, 118, 121, 138, 146, 153, 167, 174, 178, and 192. The number of individual items in *Good Formulas* agrees with the "general number" (*zonghao*) that Hu Daojing gave to Bao Tingbo's (1728–1814) edition of *Su's and Shen's Formulas*. Bao's edition is an edited and reprinted version that Cheng Yongpei printed in 1794.

35. Items 059, 079, 088, 106, 161, 186, 188, 190, 205, and 214.

36. Items 050, 058B, 071, 072B, 093, 113, 119, 158, 167, 174, 177, 202, and 209.

37. Items 058A, 058B, 068, 071, 075, 078, 082, 083, 085, 091, 108, 110, 113, 138, 145, 148, 151, 152, 161, 170, 180, 196, 206, 215, 216, 218, 227, and 231.

38. Items 063, 084, 090, 175, 176, 179b, 193, 195, 203, 213, and 224.

39. Items 051, 060, 072A, 073–075, 077, 078, 082, 087, 092, 093, 096, 097, 099–101, 106, 107, 109, 110, 115–17, 120, 132, 138, 145–47, 149, 154–56, 163, 164, 168, 171, 183, 191, 192, 200, 204, 209, 211, 212, 216, 220, 222, 224, 226, and 234h.

40. Item 205.

41. Items 234a–234g.

42. *Shen Kuo quanji*, 66.681.

43. *Xu zizhi tongjian changbian*, 283.6936–37.

44. *Xu zizhi tongjian changbian*, 283.6933.

45. On hearsay as an important source of information in *Brush Talks*, see Egan, "Shen Kuo Chats."

46. The scope of the term "witness" (*mudu*) in Shen's preface encompassed both his personal experience and others' observations, a scope that contrasts sharply with our common understanding of witnessing (i.e., personally seeing something). To prevent confusion about this divergent meaning, throughout this book, whenever I refer to

Shen Kuo's phrase *mudu* in his preface, I use "witness" or a cognate of it in quotation marks.

47. For a thorough study of Shen Kuo's interests and achievements in scientific fields, see Sivin, "Shen Kua."

48. For a list of examples of how Shen Kuo is received in contemporary China, see Zuo, *Shen Gua's Empiricism*, 1–4.

49. *Xinjiaozheng mengxi bitan*, 7.78. For a discussion of the relationship between the intricate number and degree and of the relationship between particular things and deep orders in *Brush Talks*, see Zuo, *Shen Gua's Empiricism*, 76–98.

50. *Xinjiaozheng mengxi bitan*, 7.85–86.

51. For a discussion of Shen's activities in these projects, see Zuo, *Shen Gua's Empiricism*, 56–75.

52. *Shen Kuo quanji*, 28.179.

53. For a survey of textual techniques that were used to facilitate the retrieval of information in formularies before and during the Song era, see Ruth Yun-ju Chen, "Quest for Efficiency."

54. For an overview of medical innovations in the Song, see Miyashita Saburō, "Sō Gen no iryō"; and Goldschmidt, *Evolution of Chinese Medicine*.

55. For the formation of the premise that governance was based on benevolence in the Song era, see Hartman, *Making of Song Dynasty History*, 248–73.

56. Hinrichs, "Song and Jin Periods"; Smith, *Forgotten Disease*, 67–84.

57. Li Jingwei, "Bei Song huangdi yu yixue." The body of scholarship on Song emperors' interest in medicine is too vast to be comprehensively cited here. In this scholarship, Li Jingwei's important pioneering study lists 284 edicts pertaining to medicine that the Northern Song emperors issued.

58. The estimation of five formularies is drawn from Hinrichs, "Governance through Medical Texts," 218. The estimation of twenty-five in the Song era is drawn from Ruth Yun-ju Chen, "Songdai shidafu canyu difang yishu kanyin xintan." To be more specific, of the twenty-five medical texts, ten were completed before the Song dynasty but were edited by the Song court, two were formularies first privately written by Song officials and then submitted to the court, and thirteen were compiled by the Song court itself.

59. For more on medical governance as an innovation in Song medicine, see Hinrichs, "Medical Transforming of Governance," "Governance through Medical Texts," and *Shamans, Witchcraft, and Quarantine*. For statistics of printed editions of medical literature during the Song dynasty, see Ruth Yun-ju Chen, "Songdai shidafu canyu difang yishu kanyin xintan." Of course, in addition to medicine, religious therapies were popular among the general public and scholar-officials in the Song era; see Sivin, *Health Care*, 93–182.

60. Kurz has suggested that the projects designed to compile encyclopedic works

that Emperor Taizong ordered served as a means of integrating cultural elites from recently conquered southern regions into the new Song regime. Kurz, "Politics of Collecting Knowledge."

61. For more on the differences between *The Imperial Grace Formulary* and *The Formulary for Magnificent Healing and Universal Relief* in terms of their compilation purposes and transmission, see Fan, *Bei Song jiaozheng yishuju xintan*, 35–57.

62. Hinrichs and Hong, "Unwritten Life (and Death)"; Han, *Songdai yixue fangshu de xingcheng yu chuanbo yingyong yanjiu*, 83–156.

63. For a detailed English-language discussion of the early Northern Song's effort to reunite China, see Lorge, *Reunification of China*.

64. On scholar-officials interested in medicine during the Song period, see Chen Yuan-peng, *Liang Song de "shangyi shiren" yu "ruyi."*

65. For more on changes in the availability of the directorate's medical imprints in the Northern Song period see Fan, *Bei Song jiaozheng yishuju xintan*, 191–200.

66. Cherniack, "Book Culture," 43–45.

67. On the growing number of self-taught medical learners since the twelfth century, see Leung, "Medical Learning," 374–98.

68. On tactile perception and pulse diagnosis in early China, see Hsu, *Pulse Diagnosis*.

69. Chen Yuan-peng, "Songdai ruyi," 278–80.

70. Dong, *Lüshe beiyao fang*, 2.

71. For a thorough analysis of the remedies in *The Formulary for Travel Houses*, see Wu, "Daoting tushuo zhihou."

72. Chaffee, *Thorny Gates of Learning*, 35.

73. For an articulation of why the notions "professional" and "specialist" fail to describe Song physicians as an occupation, see Sivin, *Health Care*, 76–77.

74. On being self-taught as a new model of medical transmission owing to the popularization of printing, see Leung, "Medical Learning," 391–93.

75. On how the abundance of books (in both print and manuscript form) changed reading cultures and the composition of poems and historiographies in the late Northern Song era, see Egan, "To Count Grains," 33–52; and Yugen Wang, *Ten Thousand Scrolls*, 174–94.

76. *Xu zizhi tongjian changbian*, 186.4487.

77. Fan Ka Wai analyzed this memorandum in detail, arguing that Han Qi's suggestion was part of his long-term effort to increase the availability of medical resources for residents and soldiers who lived in the northwestern frontier of Song China. Fan, *Bei Song jiaozheng yishuju xintan*, 15–17.

78. For a study of the correlation between the period when the bureau was established between 1057 and 1069 and the spike in recorded epidemics between 1041 and

1060, see Goldschmidt, *Evolution of Chinese Medicine*, 77–95. Fan Ka Wai has challenged Goldschimidt's observation. See Fan, "Songdai yixue fazhan de waiyuan yinsu."

79. For an English-language discussion of the bureau's founding and history as well as its influence on the development of Song medicine, see Goldschmidt, *Evolution of Chinese Medicine*.

80. Ban, *Han shu*, 30.1701. For a discussion of the significance of *Seven Catalogs* in terms of early Chinese historiographies that recorded healers, see Brown, *Art of Medicine in Early China*, 89–109.

81. "Academies and institutes" refer collectively to institutes in the central government that were dedicated to storing and editing books. Those included the Institute for the Glorification of Literature (Zhaowen Guan), the Historiography Institute (Shi Guan), and the Academy of Scholarly Worthies (Jixian Guan).

82. For an analysis of how and why the eleventh-century court-officials' advocacy of assigning officials from academies and institutes to lead text-compilation projects, see Fan, *Bei Song jiaozheng yishuju xintan*, 22–34.

83. For examples of the procedure, see Fan, *Bei Song jiaozheng yishuju xintan*, 95–163.

84. Qian, *Song ben Shanghan lun wenxian shilun*, 5.

85. *Su weigong wenji*, 65.999.

86. Gao Baoheng, "Jiaoding *Beiji qianjin yaofang* houxu," in *Beiji qianjin yaofang*, 7.

87. *Su weigong wenji*, 65.999.

88. Qian, *Song ben Shanghan lun wenxian shilun*, 5.

89. Sun Zhao, "Jiaozheng *Waitai miyao fang* xu," in *Waitai miyao fang*, 1.

90. The foregoing analysis of the four prefaces that officials in the bureau wrote to *Essential Formulas* does not mean that they always shared the same criteria for the quality of medical treatises. For the heterogeneity among the officials in the bureau, especially in terms of their medical background and bureaucratic positions, see Fan, *Bei Song jiaozheng yishuju xintan*, 67–94.

91. *Shen Kuo quanji*, 66.678. Shen Kuo knew that the bureau had edited *The Imperial Library Formulary*, given that he mentioned the Yellow Dragon Decoction formula that came from the bureau edition.

92. In the Song era, imprints that the Directorate of Education issued were criticized by many scholar-officials, including for the "typographical" errors they found in the imprints. See Cherniack, "Book Culture and Textual Transmission in Sung China," 57–67. Yi Sumei compared the dosages of ingredients in Shen's formulas that *Su's and Shen's Formulas* collected with those in formulas that listed the same ingredients but were collected in formularies that the Song court compiled or edited. The comparison shows a divergence of dosages between the two. This, Yi proposed, suggests that Shen

did not trust the court-commissioned versions of formulas. See Yi, "Songdai de shiren yu yifang," 90–91.

93. Dean-Jones, "*Autopsia, Historia,*" 42.

94. Pomata, "Word of the Empirics."

95. Zuo, *Shen Gua's Empiricism*, 229.

96. Scholarship on the history of science and medicine revealed how modes of reasoning were firmly situated in the political, social, and institutional contexts of a given culture. For instance, for scholarship on this topic in ancient China and Greece, see Lloyd and Sivin, *Way and the Word*; for scholarship on early modern Europe, see Shapin and Schaffer, *Leviathan and the Air-Pump*.

TWO Textual Claims and Local Investigations

1. See, for example, Métailié, "Lun Songdai bencao yu bowuxue zhuzuo zhongde lixue 'gewu' guan," 295–97. In this chapter, I argue that the trend toward documenting authors' local investigations and medical policies during Emperor Huizong's regime played a more significant role than the neo-Confucian concept did in the production of *Elucidating the Meaning*. Paul Unschuld has said only that empirical verification was a feature of *Elucidating the Meaning*. He was more interested in examining the manual as a watershed in the history of pharmacology in China, because for the first time there was a source that integrated pragmatic use of drugs into systematic theories of cosmological correspondence. See Unschuld, *Medicine in China: A History of Pharmaceutics*, 100. Georges Métailié has compared pre-sixteenth-century Chinese pharmacological texts, including *Elucidating the Meaning*, to pre-sixteenth-century European pharmacological texts. See Métailié, *Science and Civilisation in China*, 116–17.

2. *Junzhai dushuzhi jiaozheng*, 9.384.

3. *Bencao yanyi*, 4.21; 5.35; 6.38, 41; 7.50; 12.72; 13.79, 81; 15.95; 17.125; 20.147. Kou served as an "official in charge of documents in the county office" (*zhubu*) in Wucheng County in En Prefecture (Hebei) in 1077. See *Xu zizhi tongjian changbian*, 283.6930.

4. For acclaimed English-language scholarship on Tao's life, see Strickmann, "On the Alchemy."

5. For important textual sources for the compilation of *Jiayou Materia Medica* and *Illustrated Materia Medica*, see Fan, *Bei Song jiaozheng yishuju xintan*, 120–43.

6. Pharmacological encyclopedias lost state patronage under the Ming and Qing dynasties. On this shift, see Bian, *Know Your Remedies*.

7. *Bencao yanyi*, 1.2.

8. *Bencao shiyi jishi*, 9.408.

9. For statistics regarding sources of information in Tao's work, see Chen Yuan-peng, "*Bencaojing jizhu* suozai 'Tao zhu.'"

NOTES TO PAGES 42–47   *163*

10. Okanishi, *Honzō gaisetsu*, 151. Okanishi also noticed the informal style of *Elucidating the Meaning*. In this chapter, in addition to noting the informality of its style, I explain why Kou Zongshi chose it.

11. *Bencao yanyi*, 16.104.

12. A style name is a name gave to an individual upon reaching adulthood as an addition to, rather than a replacement for, one's given name. Adults of the same generation would use style names, instead of given names, to refer to one another.

13. *Bencao yanyi*, 16.113. Translation is adapted from Unschuld, *Medicine in China: A History of Pharmaceutics*, 100–101.

14. *Bencaojing jizhu*, 6.449.

15. On medical subgenres with distinct epistemic orientations, see Pomata, "Medical Case Narrative." On genre-blending in Ming pharmacological texts, see Bian, *Know Your Remedies*, 40–44.

16. Miyashita ("Sō Gen no iryō," 186) suggested this possible scenario.

17. Over the past five decades, English-speaking scholars have long debated translations of *li* in Chinese thought, especially in neo-Confucianism, rendering it as "reason," "law," "principle," "pattern," and "coherence," in addition to several other choices. For a recent and critical review of these translations, see Ziporyn, "Form, Principle, Pattern, or Coherence?" Peterson rendered *li* as "coherence" to suggest that it is "the quality or characteristic of sticking together." Adopting his translation, Bol indicates that in many instances in neo-Confucianism, *li* was used as a descriptive term referring to how things worked and also as a normative term "for identifying how things should work." I shall compare differences between Kou's understanding of *li* and the Northern Song neo-Confucianists' other claims regarding *li* later in the next section. See Peterson, "Another Look at *Li*"; Bol, *Neo-Confucianism in History*, 162–63.

18. *Kaibao bencao (jifu ben)*, 3.103. Actually, the relationship between "jade spring water" and "jade-thick fluid" had already been addressed in *Kaibao Materia Medica*, which was completed by the Song court in 974 but remains only in scattered and fragmented entries. *Kaibao Materia Medica* remarked that *Thirty-Six Methods of Water* (Sanshiliu shuifa) of *The Transcendent Canon* (Xianjing) used "jade spring water" in reference to a "jade-thick fluid" that was transformed from jade.

19. *Bencao yanyi*, 8.53.

20. *Bencao yanyi*, 16.107.

21. *Bencao yanyi*, 6.40–41.

22. For an excellent new study of how authors of pharmacological works in China between the fifth and seventh centuries discussed pronunciation and flavors of medicinal substances, see Chen Hao, *Shenfen xushi yu zhishi biaoshu zhijian de yizhe zhiyi*, 303–46. As shown in Chen Hao's study, authors' sensory perceptions of the taste of a given substance by no means served as the only factor determining its "flavors"; textual

records about substances that were drawn from earlier classics sometimes played more significant roles in those authors' determinations.

23. For further analysis of the format in which *Illustrated Materia Medica* presented information, see Chen Yuan-peng, "Zhongyaocai niuhuang de shengchanlishi jiqi bencaoyaotu suosheji de zhishijiegou."

24. *Bencao yanyi*, 1.14.

25. *Er Cheng ji*, "*Yishu*," 18.188, 193; 22. 277; Graham, *Two Chinese Philosophers*; Bol, "Reconceptualizing the Order," 716–20. On Northern Song thinkers' varying opinions of the meaning of the terms "investigating things" (*gewu*) and "attaining knowledge" (*zhizhi*) and on the relationships between the two terms, see Le, *Zhuzi gewu zhizhilun yanjiu*, 9–35.

26. Despite the fact that the *li* Kou mentioned did not link to the ultimate and unitary coherence of the universe, I still choose to translate it as "coherence" to highlight his emphasis on the perfect match between an object or affair and its linguistic expression.

27. Furth, "Physician as Philosopher."

28. For recent studies of the trend toward accounting for authors' empirical verification in notebooks completed in the Song, see Zuo, *Shen Gua's Empiricism*; and Ellen Cong Zhang, "To Be 'Erudite.'" The appearance of botanical treatises in the eleventh century that described horticulture and the connoisseurship of floral beauty reflects another indication of Song scholar-officials' growing attention to hands-on knowledge. See Egan, *Problem of Beauty*, 109–61. On the travel accounts in the Song, see Hargett, *Jade Mountains*, 90–121. For authors' empirical observation of objects in inventories of things, see Siebert, "Animals as Text"; and Mai, "Double Life."

29. I elaborate on the trend below with the caveat that not every work discussed in this section was composed with the singular goal of verifying regional phenomena, nor did their authors share the same perceptions of the relationship between the substances or affairs they investigated and *li* (coherence).

30. This combination of book learning and empirical investigations is reminiscent of what scholars have called "learned empiricism" in early modern Europe. For more on learned empiricism, see Pomata and Siraisi, "Introduction," 17–28.

31. Yu Xin and Zhong Wumou have pointed out this trend. In addition to sharing their observations, in this chapter I shall take their findings a step further by placing this trend in the context of the long-term development of the empirical strategy in middle-period China. See Yu and Zhong, "Bowuxue de zhongwan Tang tujing," 333–35. For the classic study on the Tang understanding of the south, see Schafer, *Vermilion Bird*.

32. *Jiu Tang shu*, 38.1384.

33. *Jiu Tang shu*, 40.1598, 1601.

34. For shifts in geographical areas that the term "Lingnan" covered, see Ma Lei, "Lingnan, Wuling kao."

35. *Erya, zhong*, 133.

36. *Erya shu*, 47.

37. On places in Lingnan where Duan lived, see Suzuki, "Dan Kōro sen *Hokutoroku* ni tsuite."

38. *Beihu lu*, 1.523, 525–30; 2.534, 536–38, 543–44.

39. On the basis of the titles of books in this literature that those later works cited, twenty-two known titles that included "records of exceptional things" existed between the Han and Tang dynasties. For the list, see Wang Jingbo, "Han Tang jian yiyi *Yiwu zhi* kaoshu." Wang Jingbo (in "Cong dili bowu zaji dao zhiguai chuanqi") suggested that entries in the corpus before the Tang era are based in part on authors' observations. On my reading of his article, however, he seems to count any description of local affairs as more or less an example of an author's witness. In the same article, Wang also proposed that, from a modern perspective, works in the literature of Tang China eventually paid more attention to literary entertainment, such as accounts of extraordinary events, than to factual information on specific regions, such as descriptions of local plants.

40. On the "records of exceptional things" literature as part of the development of local writing between the third and seventh centuries, see Chittick, "Development of Local Writing."

41. *Beihu lu*, 1.523.

42. *Beihu lu*, 1.524.

43. For examples of authors' firsthand experience in Liu Xun's and Fang Qianli's works, see Yu and Zhong, "Bowuxue de zhongwan Tang tujing," 335–36. Liu lived in Guang Prefecture (in Guangdong) sometime between 896 and 904. On Fang Qianli's official career and his work, see Wang Chengwen, "Tangdai Fang Qianli ji qi *Touhuang zalu* kaozheng."

44. For an English-language discussion of *Miscellaneous Morsels*, especially Duan Chengshi's personal element and first-person narratives in the work, see Reed, "Motivation and Meaning."

45. *Youyang zazu jiaojian*, 17.1241.

46. *Youyang zazu jiaojian*, 17.1249.

47. Zou, *Tang Wudai biji yanjiu*. Zou Fuqing has found only three notebooks (including *Northward-Facing Doors*) in the Tang and Five Dynasties eras whose authors asked others to write prefaces.

48. See Lu Xisheng, "*Beihu lu* xu," in *Beihu lu*, 519.

49. For a discussion of two hundred texts that Duan Gonglu cited in *Northward-Facing Doors*, see Yu and Zhong, "Bowuxue de zhongwan Tang tujing," 315–24.

50. For recent studies on the popularity of tales in the late Tang period, see Allen, *Shifting Stories*.

51. The translation is from Allen, *Shifting Stories*, 1.

52. Lu Xisheng, "*Beihu lu* xu," in *Beihu lu*, 519.

53. In the primary sources I have encountered, the term *bowu* referred before the Song era to intellectual practices associated with knowing things broadly rather than to the discipline that we know today as natural history. For a discussion of how practices changed within natural history in late imperial China, see Elman, *On Their Own Terms*, 43–46.

54. Pomata, "Observation Rising."

55. Zuo, *Shen Gua's Empiricism*, 193–95, 229–30.

56. Fang Rui, *Sun Guangxian yu Beimeng suoyan yanjiu*, 134–38; *Beimeng suoyan*, 256. Fang indicated that the accounts of Sun Guangxian's personal experience occupied a substantial portion of *Northern Dreams*.

57. *Taiping guangji*, 479.3945.

58. While both *Miscellaneous Morsels from Youyang* and *Brush Talks* exhibited an empirical approach to received information, Fu's research has insightfully noted that Shen Kuo in *Brush Talks* adapted entries on divine marvels and strange occurrences from *Miscellaneous Morsels* and reformulated them into more secular terms. See Fu, "Contextual and Taxonomic Study."

59. *Xinjiaozheng mengxi bitan*, 20.197; 21.209, 219.

60. *Xinjiaozheng mengxi bitan*, 16.166.

61. Aoyama has indicated that the Song era witnessed the popular practice in which scholar-officials critically examined and verified information in the "map guide" (*tujing*) genre. See Aoyama, *Tō Sō Jidai No KōTsū to Chishi Chizu No Kenkyū*, 490–91.

62. *Mingdao zazhi*, 18. The translation is based on Bol's translation ("Literati Miscellany," 148–49).

63. For a full translation of this account and its groundbreaking role in the development of travel accounts, see Hargett, "Travel Records," 388–91. On Su Shi's other innovations in travel literature, see Hargett, "What Need Is There."

64. *Su Shi wenji*, 11.371.

65. For Song scholar-officials' view of travel as a means of pursuing knowledge and improving their scholarship, see Ellen Cong Zhang, *Transformative Journeys*, 162–67. For travel cultures in Song China, see Ihara, *Sōdai Chūgoku o tabisuru*.

66. Hargett, "Song Dynasty Local Gazetteers," 417–24.

67. On the flourishing of notebooks as the primary mode of a new literati culture under the Song, for example, see Bol, "Literati Miscellany."

68. *Xinjiaozheng mengxi bitan*, 26.262–71.

69. Zuo's recent monograph on *Brush Talks* demonstrates that this notebook was

Shen's last intellectual expression of his view of an ideal way of learning. See Zuo, *Shen Gua's Empiricism*.

70. According to Liu's monograph, *Approaching Correctness* is the most frequently cited title among Tang pharmacological texts. See Liu Yan, *Healing with Poisons*, 95. On botanical knowledge in *Approaching Correctness*, see Métailié, *Science and Civilisation*, 48–56.

71. *Bencao yanyi*, 7.47–49; 9.59–60; 11.71; 13.82; *Xinjiaozheng mengxi bitan*, 26.267, 270–71.

72. *Bencao yanyi*, 9.59; 11.71; *Xinjiaozheng mengxi bitan*, 26.270–71.

73. My understanding of features and *li* in *Brush Talks* relies to a great extent on Zuo, *Shen Gua's Empiricism*, 169–200.

74. *Song huiyao jigao*, 8290–91.

75. Wang Jiakui, "Yanzhi jingyi," 69–70.

76. On the general translation of the opening section of *Elucidating the Meaning*, see Unschuld, *Medicine in China*, 86–89.

77. *Bencao yanyi*, 1.2.

78. *Bencao yanyi*, 1.2.

79. Huizong had been regarded as a decadent ruler who was chiefly responsible for the fall of Northern Song China, the most advanced state in the twelfth-century world. Recent studies have modified this view, recasting him as a ruler of great ambition who aspired to launch numerous political reforms, cultural projects, and social welfare programs. For more on this new view, see seminal essays collected in Ebrey and Bickford eds., *Emperor Huizong*; and Ebrey, *Emperor Huizong*.

80. *Song huiyao jigao*, 2793.

81. In addition to running medical academies, the Song court also operated other technical schools, such as military academies. On the development of technical schools under the directorate in the Song, see Thomas H. C. Lee, *Government Education*, 91–103.

82. On the emergence and development of "scholar-physicians" in the Song and Yuan dynasties, see, for instance, Hymes, "Not Quite Gentlemen?"; Chen Yuan-peng, *Liang Song de "shangyi shiren" yu "ruyi"*; and Chu, "Song-Ming zhiji de yishi yu 'ruyi.'"

83. *Song shi*, 21.394.

84. *Bencao yanyi*, 1.2.

85. *Song huiyao jigao*, 2801–2. Between 1103 and 1120, the medical academy in the capital was abolished and reestablished three times. On detailed discussion of medical policies under Huizong's reign, see Goldschmidt, "Huizong's Impact on Medicine"; and Fan, *Bei Song jiaozheng yishuju xintan*, 259–306.

86. I will discuss Zhu's formulary at greater length in chapter 3.

87. On Zhu Gong's submission and return to officialdom, see Fan, *Bei Song jiaozheng yishuju xintan*, 304–6.

88. *Song da zhaoling ji*, 219.843.

89. On the legal weight of "imperial brush hand-drafted edicts" under the Song, see Tokunaga, "Sōdai no gyohitsu shushō." Fang Chengfeng's recent research argues against an earlier view that the imperial brush during Huizong's reign bypassed the bureaucratic process that produced and promulgated general edicts, such as ministerial consultation. See Fang Chengfeng, "Yubi, yubi shouzhao, yu Bei Song Huizong chao de tongzhi fangshi."

90. For a full translation of this edict and compilation process of *Jiayou Materia Medica* and *Illustrated Materia Medica*, see Goldschmidt, *Evolution of Chinese Medicine*, 111–15.

91. *Song huiyao jigao*, 2793.

92. *Bencao yanyi*, 1.2.

93. *Bencao yanyi*. 1.2. I added the numbers for convenience to inform the discussion that follows.

94. *Bencao yanyi*, 1.3.

95. See "Fu Kou Zongshi zha," in *Bencao yanyi*, appendix, 153. On the establishment of the Institution for Collecting and Purchasing Drugs, see Chen Cheng, "Jin biao," in *Zengguang taiping huimin hejiju jufang*, 3.

96. The number and scope of the texts cited in *Validated and Classified* is based on Zhou, *Zhenglei bencao yu Songdai xueshu wenhua yanjiu*, 76, 208–23.

97. On the compilation of *Validated and Classified*, see Shang, "Tang Shenwei *Zhenglei bencao* yange," 3–4.

98. Zhou, *Zhenglei bencao yu Songdai xueshu wenhua yanjiu*, 38–54. Before 1108, *Validated and Classified* had already been printed privately. The textual history of this collection has been the subject of intensive scholarly debate. For a classic Japanese-language study on this topic, see Watanabe, "Tō Shinbi no Kēshi shōrui bikyū honzō no kētō to sono hanpon." Reviewing and revising earlier Japanese- and Chinese-language studies, Zhou provided a new history. My understanding of the textual history is based on Zhou's research.

99. Fan, *Bei Song jiaozheng yishuju xintan*, 264–65. As the historian Fan Ka Wai has observed, this assignment conflicted with a conventional policy in which the Northern Song court commissioned "Confucian officials" (*ruchen*) to lead the project of editing medical treatises, even though Cao Xiaozhong claimed that his editing methods followed those they set up.

100. Beijing Tushuguan, ed., *Zhongguo banke tulu*, vol. 1, 30.

101. Okanishi, *Song yiqian yiji kao*, 1224.

NOTES TO PAGES 67–72

102. On further information about this integrated version, see Chen Xiaolan, "Xinbian leiyao tuzhu bencao jiqi chuankeben kaocha."

103. On the book printing in Jianyang in imperial China, see Chia, *Printing for Profit*.

104. *Xinbian furen daquan liangfang*, 20.13b, 14a. It should be noted that its author, Chen Ziming, attributed this medical case and formula to a famous Southern Song physician, Chen Yan. For other examples, see *Yishuo*, 9.31b.

105. See, for instance, *Yungu zaji*, 1.16; and *Yan fanlu xuji*, 5.221.

106. *Zhizhai shulu jieti*, 13.386.

107. Bian, "Ever-Expanding Pharmacy," 311–13.

THREE Demonstration of Medical Virtuosity

In this chapter, my translations of Xu Shuwei's cold damage disorder cases are all based on Goldschmidt, *Medical Practice in Twelfth-Century China*, which provides full translations and thorough annotations of the medical cases in *Ninety Discussions*, a work attributed to Xu. Note that rhubarb is an ingredient in the decoction Xu wanted to administer in the opening case narrative.

1. For a comparison of the various versions of the story, see Ruth Yun-ju Chen, "Songdai shidafu canyu difang yishu kanyin xintan." The versions discussed in Chen's article meanwhile also include several versions of the notion that Xu Shuwei's father also practiced medicine. The most reliable source of information about Xu's father is Xu Shuwei's own preface to *The Formulary with Explanatory Historical Context*. The preface, on my reading, implies that his father was not a physician.

2. *Puji benshifang*, 83.

3. Hong Mai, *Yijian zhi, jia zhi*, 5.38.

4. Lee Jen-der, "Han Tang zhijian jiating zhongde jiankang zhaogu yu xingbie," 29–32; Chen Hao, *Shenfen xushi yu zhishi biaoshu zhijian de yizhe zhiyi*, 87–130.

5. Chen Yuan-peng, *Liang Song de "shangyi shiren" yu "ruyi,"* 45–112; Yu Xinzhong, "'Liangyi liangxiang.'"

6. Goldschmidt, *Evolution of Chinese Medicine*, 19–41. Differing from Goldschmidt's claim, Fan Ka Wai's observation indicates that the imperial patronage already appeared in the Tang. See Fan, *Dayi jingcheng*, 73–125.

7. Hymes, "Not Quite Gentlemen?" Cases that Hymes cited about classically educated men practicing medicine as an occupation mostly occur during the Yuan dynasty, when the Mongol court closed down the civil service examination over fifty years but valued medicine as practical knowledge. Chen Yuan-peng found more instances in the Song era in which candidates who repeatedly failed turned to healing people to maintain their livelihood. See Chen Yuan-peng, "Songdai ruyi."

8. On Zhen Prefecture as a transfer port in the Song, see Liang, "Cong nanbei dao dongxi."

9. On Zhang Yu's activities, see Huang Kuan-chung, *Nan Song shidai kang Jin de yijun*, 88.

10. Zhang Yan, "*Puji benshifang* xu," in *Xuxiu Siku quanshu shanghan lei yizhu jicheng*, vol. 1, 602.

11. *Baoqing bencao zhezhong*, 3.468.

12. *Song huiyao jigao*, 20.5637.

13. See Zhang Yan, "*Puji benshifang* xu," in *Xuxiu Siku quanshu shanghan lei yizhu jicheng*, vol. 1, 602.

14. *Yunzhuang ji*, 4.105–6. Historians disagree on the year when Xu was the academician of the Hanlin Academy. Li Zhizhong proposed the year 1135. However, Zhang Haipeng's research notes that, according to Zeng Xie's 1173 preface to Xu's *Formulary with Explanatory Historical Context*, Xu was only a staff member assisting the magistrate of Hui Prefecture in 1136. Considering that the rank of assistant staff member was much lower than the rank of academician of the Hanlin Academy, Zhang proposed that it was likely that Xu served as an assistant staff member before being appointed academician. If that were the case, Zhang indicates, the year when Xu was the academician would have been later than 1136. See Li Zhizhong, "Yuan kan Xu Shuwei *Shanghan baizheng ge* yu *Shanghan fawei lun*"; Zhang Haipeng, "Xu Shuwei yizhu zai Nan Song de kanke yu liuchuan," 307.

15. For further details of Xu's life, see Goldschmidt, *Medical Practice*, 12–16. Goldschmidt, without citing concrete evidence, suggests that Xu retired over his disagreement with the death sentence that the court imposed on Yue Fei, the powerful general and loyal supporter of the Song empire.

16. These six treatise titles can be found in the preface to the Yuan-dynasty edition of *Shanghan baizheng ge*, which is kept in the National Central Library in Taiwan. It has no page numbers.

17. The date is based on the latest date recorded in Xu's cases in this treatise.

18. *Lou Yue ji*, 50.945.

19. *Baoqing bencao zhezhong*, 3.468.

20. Han and Yu, "Nan Song Xu Shuwei yian yu linchuang jibing zheliao chutan," 1. Other studies that consider Xu Shuwei to be the author of *Ninety Discussions*, for instance, include, Ye, *Shanghan xueshu shi*, 295; Goldschmidt, "Reasoning with Cases" and *Medical Practice*; and Lu, *Songdai shanghan xueshu yu wenxian kaolun*, 200.

21. *Yongle dadian*, 3614.2176, 2179.

22. *Puji benshifang*, 8.144.

23. *Shanghan jiushi lun*, 58. Goldschmidt noticed this difference but did not use it to question the authorship of *Ninety Discussions*. See Goldschmidt, *Medical Practice*, 39.

24. *Nan shi*, 57.1420.

25. *Nan shi*, 6.168. On the eight companions of the prince of the Jingling, see Tian, *Beacon Fire*, 19–20.

26. Lu, *Songdai shanghan xueshu yu wenxian kaolun*, 202–4.

27. For the recent study of the printing of *The Formulary with Explanatory Historical Contexts*, see Ruth Yun-ju Chen, "Songdai shidafu canyu difang yishu kanyin xintan," 450–52, 484–86, 490.

28. *Puji benshifang*, 7.137.

29. *Puji benshifang*, preface, 83.

30. For a recent study of Meng Qi and his *Poems with Explanatory Historical Contexts*, see Liu Ning, "'Shihua' yu 'benshi' zaitan"; and Yu Cailin, *Tangshi benshi yanjiu*.

31. On the composition and circulation of *Lyrics with Explanatory Historical Contexts*, see Zhu, "*Shixian benshi quzi ji* xin kaoding."

32. Goldschmidt noticed that the formulary title is based on *Poems with Explanatory Historical Contexts* as well, but he concluded that "the meaning is not parallel." Goldschmidt, *Medical Practice*, 18.

33. *Benshi shi*, 4.

34. *Benshi shi*, 4.

35. *Puji benshifang*, preface, 83.

36. *Benshi shi*, 4.

37. *Xiaoer yaozheng zhijue*, preface, 3.

38. Hsiung, "Facts in the Tale."

39. The number of such medical treatises completed before the Song dynasty is based on Ye, *Shanghan xueshu shi*, 288–91. The number of Song medical treatises comes from Lu, *Songdai shanghan xueshu yu wenxian kaolun*.

40. Goldschmidt, *Evolution of Chinese Medicine*, 69–102.

41. Fan, "Songdai yixue fazhan de waiyuan yinsu," 332. For other explanations, see Despeux, "System"; and Fan, *Bei Song Jiaozheng yishuju xintan*, 68–80.

42. *Shanghan lun*, preface, 5.

43. Qian, "*Shanghan lun*" wenxian xinkao, 9–12. For instance, some studies have proposed that the term *jian'an* in the preface was mistranscribed from the term *jianning*, as severe epidemics took place during the Jianning reign (168–172).

44. For a recent review of and discussion about the authorship and accuracy of the preface, Zhang Ji's life and career, and changes in Zhang's persona from the third to the thirteenth centuries, see Brown, *Art of Medicine*, 110–29.

45. This received view can be seen in Unschuld, *Medicine in China: A History of Ideas*, 168–69; Ye, *Shanghan xueshushi*, 5; and Sivin, *Health Care*, 56, 63.

46. Goldschmidt, *Evolution of Chinese Medicine*, 137–72.

47. Boyanton, "*Treatise on Cold Damage*," 19–54. Boyanton additionally has ob-

served that in the eleventh century, the dissemination of *Treatise on Cold Damage* encouraged a new phenomenon, that is, when medical authors discussed cold damage medicine, they focused on Zhang Ji's works. Boyanton called this phenomenon the "narrowing of vision" of cold damage medicine and the "broadening of discourse" on Zhang's texts.

48. Ma Jixing, *Zhongyi wenxian xue*, 117–23; Qian, *"Shanghan lun" wenxian tongkao*, 123, and *"Shanghan lun" wenxian xinkao*, 255–56.

49. Qian, *"Shanghan lun" wenxian xinkao*, 91.

50. *Xu zizhi tongjian changbian*, 335.8084–85.

51. Lu, *Songdai shanghan xueshu yu wenxian kaolun*, 252–53.

52. *Nanyang huoren shu*, 5.

53. *Nanyang huoren shu*, 5; Li Bao, "Ti *Beishan jiujing* hou," in *Beishan jiujing*, 834.

54. *Quan Song wen*, 2970.229–30.

55. *Nanyang huoren shu*, preface, 6.

56. *Nanyang huoren shu*, 7; *Yifang leiju*, 32.136.

57. *Nanyang huoren shu*, 7.

58. *Yijing zhengbenshu*, 358.

59. Lu, *Songdai shanghan xueshu yu wenxian kaolun*, 29–51.

60. Brown, *Art of Medicine*, 125.

61. Goldschmidt, "Reasoning with Cases."

62. Lu, *Songdai shanghan xueshu yu wenxian kaolun*, 54–57.

63. The term *xue* is translated as "blood." However, this term means more than the red liquid flowing through the bodies of humans and animals in the modern Western sense. *Xue* in classical Chinese medicine additionally meant the yin vitalities of the body, as a counterpart to the yang vitalities of the qi of the body.

64. *Puji benshifang*, 8.144.

65. *Puji benshifang*, 9.152–53. The translation is based on Goldschmidt, *Medical Practice*, 287–89.

66. Unschuld suggests that some sources in the extant *Inner Canon* could date from the Han era. Keegan regards the extant *Inner Canon* as having been included in a series of compilations within the Yellow Emperor medical tradition during the Han and Tang dynasties. Other studies point out that the Northern Song court edited *Inner Canon* extensively in 1026/1027 and 1067. See Sivin, *"Huang ti nei ching"*; Unschuld, *Huang di nei jing Suwen*, 3–5; and Keegan, *"Huang-ti nei-ching."*

67. Boyanton has likewise suspected that Xu's debates with physicians on his cases "were embellished or invented by Xu to suit his purposes," which, in Boyanton's reading, include "self-promotion, instruction, doctrinal polemics, clinical innovation, or even exegesis." Boyanton, "Hermeneutics."

68. *Puji benshifang*, 8.143.

69. *Nanyang huoren shu*, 6.

70. *Puji benshifang*, 9.152.

71. *Puji benshifang*, 9.153.

72. *Puji benshifang*, 8.146.

73. *Puji benshifang*, 8.147.

74. Lee Jen-der, "Juejing de lishi yanjiu," 206–7.

FOUR Search for Therapies in the Far South

1. This formulary is recorded under an alternative name, *Treatise on Zhang* [Miasma] (Zhanglun), in the standard history *History of the Song Dynasty*. In its extant version, it is entitled *Zhangnüe lun. Song shi*, 207.5315.

2. For the classic study on disorders in Lingnan in middle-period China, see Hsiao, "Han Song jian wenxian suojian gudai Zhongguo nanfang de dilihuangjing."

3. For this observation on the appearance of the character for *zhang*, see Zuo Peng, "Han-Tang shiqi de *zhang* yu *zhang* yixiang," 258.

4. *Hou Han shu*, 24.846.

5. *Hou Han shu*, 24.840.

6. *Hou Han shu*, 48.1598.

7. Zhang Kefeng, "Cong zhang dao zhang." Zhang Kefeng explains in part why people since the Han era had so often used the character for *zhang* (miasma) in reference to the various disorders correlated with the southern environment. He suggests that this character, which is pronounced in the same way as *zhang* (obstacles), connotes that those disorders functioned as barriers to northern immigration to the south and to Chinese exploitation of the southern frontiers.

8. Gong, "2000 nian lai Zhongguo *zhang* bing fenbu bianqian de chubu yanjiu"; Zhang Kefeng, "Cong zhang dao zhang"; Fan, *Liuchao Sui Tang yixue zhi chuancheng yu zenghe*, 141–44.

9. *Zhubing yuanhou lun jiaozhu*, 10.336.

10. On the development of the concept of disorders in Lingnan in late imperial China, see Hanson, *Speaking of Epidemics*, 69–90. On how local doctors in Lingnan in the late imperial era challenged the long-standing image of Lingnan as a disorder-inducing place, see Bretelle-Establet, "Worst Environment."

11. For an example in which *zhang* is translated as "malaria," see Miyashita, "Malaria (*yao*) in Chinese Medicine." Studies that do not use the conventional translations include Bin Yang, "Zhang on Chinese Southern Frontiers"; and Ellen Cong Zhang, "Between Life and Death."

12. On further differences between the natural-realist approach and the historicalist-

conceptualist approach, see Wilson, "On the History." For examples of applying the latter approach to the history of diseases in imperial China, see Hanson, *Speaking of Epidemics*; and Smith, *Forgotten Disease*.

13. *Song shi*, 377.11654–55. Other places where Li Qiu had been an official before his time in Ying Prefecture included Chen Prefecture (in Henan) and Fang Prefecture (in Hubei).

14. *Jianyan yilai xinian yaolu*, 127.2059, 150.2412.

15. *Song shi*, 207.5315.

16. *Yingguo Aboding daxue tushuguan cang "Yongle dadian,"* 11907.5a.

17. *Jianyan yilai xinian yaolu*, 136.2189; *Song shi*, 376.11627–28.

18. Feng, *Gu fangshu jiyi*, 125–26.

19. *Jiu Tang shu*, 89.2896–97.

20. For historical contexts in which those Tang formularies appeared, see Fan, *Dayi jingcheng*, 147–68. For fragmented contents of some of those Tang formularies, see Feng, *Gu fangshu jiyi*, 125–33.

21. For studies of the government's campaigns against those customs and expansion of scholarly medicine in the south during the Song period, see Hinrichs, "Medical Transforming of Governance," "Governance through Medical Texts," and "Catchy Epidemic." For the activities of spirit mediums in the Song era, including their healing practices, see Lin, "'Jiusu' yu 'xinfeng'"; and Wong, "Wenming tuijin zhongde xianshi yu xiangxiang."

22. *Xu zizhi tongjian changbian*, 12.271.

23. *Xu zizhi tongjian changbian*, 16.349. In most cases, the verb used in reference to the action of distributing medical texts makes it difficult to discern whether the government disseminated the texts in manuscript or printed form.

24. *Xu zizhi tongjian changbian*, 33.736.

25. *Song shi*, 284.9584.

26. *Xu zizhi tongjian changbian*, 43.914.

27. *Song shi*, 7.131.

28. *Xu zizhi tongjian changbian*, 92.2122.

29. *Waitai miyao fang*, 838.

30. *Xu zizhi tongjian changbian*, 237.5776.

31. *Daoxiang ji*, 11.256.

32. For the contents of these stelae, see Huang and Tang, "Guilin shike 'yangqi tangfang' kao."

33. Di Qing, "Lun yu nanman zou," in *Yuexi wenzai*, 4.486.

34. For the late Northern Song government's management of Guangxi, see Huang Kuan-chung, "Bei Song wanqi dui Guangxi de jinglüe."

35. Li Qiu did recommend one decoction recorded in Shen Kuo's *Good Formulas*, yet he did not endorse Shen's formulary as a reliable medical treatise for treating far-southern disorders.

36. For a thorough study of the development of foot qi as a disease category from fourth-century China to modern East Asia, see Smith, *Forgotten Disease*.

37. The character *du* in imperial Chinese medicine could refer to either poison (or toxicity) or potency, depending on the context. On *du* in connection with poison and potency in Chinese knowledge about drugs, see Unschuld, *Medicine in China: A History of Pharmaceutics*, 165–66, 286; and Yan Liu, *Healing with Poisons*.

38. *Taiping shenghui fang*, 56.1733.

39. Harper, *Early Chinese Medical Literature*, 151–53. *Gu*-poisoning has attracted considerable attention from historians and anthropologists. The scholarship on it in imperial China is too vast to be cited exhaustively here. For a pioneering English-language study on *gu*-poisoning, see Feng and Shryock, "Black Magic in China." For a recent review of studies on *gu*-poisoning in imperial China, see Chen Hsiu-fen, "Shiwu, yaoshu, yu gudu" ; and Yan Liu, *Healing with Poisons*, 69–80.

40. Yu Gengzhe, *Tangdai jibing yiliao shi chutan*, 171–99.

41. *Song huiyao jigao*, 8296.

42. *Zhouhou beijifang*, 3.77.

43. Smith, *Forgotten Disease*, 35.

44. For example, *Zhouhou beijifang*, 3.77–78; and *Zhubing yuanhou lun jiaozhu*, 13.413–22.

45. *Zhubing yuanhou lun jiaozhu*, 13.413.

46. *Zhubing yuanhou lun jiaozhu*, 13.416.

47. *Taiping shenghui fang*, 45.1385.

48. *Zhubing yuanhou lun jiaozhu*, 11.355; *Taiping shenghui fang*, 52.1604.

49. Earlier scholarship has often identified *zhang* (miasma) and *nüe* (intermittent fevers) as malaria because both disorders have symptoms of intermittent chills and fever. Nevertheless, historians are increasingly hesitant to endorse this equivalence, as it risks anachronism and ignores other symptoms associated with *zhang* and *nüe* in imperial China.

50. Fan, *Dayi jingcheng*, 244–52. For example, Fan describes how members of the Tang population prevented or treated *nüe* (intermittent fevers) through Buddhist or Daoist rituals.

51. *Zhubing yuanhou lun jiaozhu*, 10.336–37.

52. The phrase *yanfang* in the Tang and Song literature usually referred to the south (but not to Lingnan only). However, neither Tang nor Song authors explained the explicit use of this term in reference to the south. It is therefore difficult for us to infer whether its use indicated that the south was frequently regarded as a direction of the

fire phase in terms of five-phase (*wuxing*) theories or because the southern land was considered to be hot, or for other reasons.

53. *Lingnan weisheng fang, shang,* 1–2.

54. It is relatively difficult to discern this emphasis in Wang Fei's extant formulary, as he more often discussed general principles for treating various types of *zhang* disorders than individuals' symptomatic and bodily particularities.

55. *Lingnan weisheng fang, shang,* 2.

56. *Lingnan weisheng fang, shang,* 2–3.

57. *Lingnan weisheng fang, shang,* 3.

58. *Lingnan weisheng fang, shang,* 4–5.

59. *Lingnan weisheng fang, shang,* 10.

60. *Lingnan weisheng fang, shang,* 4.

61. *Lingnan weisheng fang, shang,* 11–12.

62. *Lingbiao luyi jiaobu,* 22–23.

63. The expanding presence of this practice among Southern Song local gazetteers went hand in hand with the broadened functions that they could provide in this era. See Hargett, "Historiography in Southern Sung."

64. *Bencaojing jizhu,* 7.510.

65. Some Song literati attributed the idea that drinking alcohol prevented *zhang* not only to the alcohol itself but also to the raw materials from which the drinks were made. For example, Su Shi said that he drank alcohol made from cinnamon (*gui*) to prevent *zhang.* He also cited the opinion of Tao Hongjing and Sun Simiao that cinnamon could nourish and lighten the body if one consumed it over a long period of time. *Su Shi wenji,* 20.593–94.

66. *Lingnan weisheng fang, zhong,* 30–31.

67. As Hargett indicates, the multifaceted content of *Cinnamon Sea* and Fan's personal voice in this treatise together distinguish it from "classified books" (*leishu*) and local gazetteers; *Cinnamon Sea* is better understood as a compilation of notebook writings. Following Hargett's insight, I also view *Vicarious Replies* as notebook corpora. See Hargett, *Treatises of the Supervisor,* xxxi–xxxix.

68. My translation is based on Hargett, *Treatises of the Supervisor,* 133–34.

69. *Helin yulu,* 1.338.

70. For information about Zhou Qufei's life and career, see Yang Wuquan, "Jiaozhu qianyan," 1–6.

71. *Lingwai daida jiaozhu,* preface, 1.

72. *Lingnan weisheng fang, shang,* 8–9.

73. *Lingwai daida jiaozhu,* 4.152.

74. Ellen Cong Zhang, "To Be 'Erudite.'"

75. *Lingwai daida jiaozhu,* preface, 1.

NOTES TO PAGES 114–123   *177*

76. On the idea that being an active contributor of conversational material to scholar-officials' gatherings was a valued quality of successful elite men at that time, see Ellen Cong Zhang, "Things Heard."

77. For classical studies of the promotion system in the Song officialdom, see Deng, *Songdai wenguan xuanren zhidu zhucengmian (xiuding ben)*.

78. Tung, "Confronting the Job Shortage."

79. I am deeply indebted to Hinrichs's forthcoming monograph on the phenomenon of the new intertextual space that was emerging in which physicians, literati, and officials discussed medical knowledge and practices in the Southern Song era. See Hinrichs, *Shamans, Witchcraft, and Quarantine*. In addition to the application of cold damage medicines in Lingnan, another topic discussed in the Song intertextual space was enchantment disorders. On that, see Cheng, *Divine, Demonic, and Disordered*.

80. On the integration of southern deviance into the spatially synthesized cosmology of early China, see Lewis, *Construction of Space*, 189–244. On the Song government's medical campaign in the south, see Hinrichs, *Shamans, Witchcraft, and Quarantine*.

81. *Zhubing yuanhou lun jiaozhu*, 10.336–37.

82. Hanson provides an English translation and discusses this in detail with other entries about the five directions in *Basic Questions*. Hanson, *Speaking of Epidemics*, 30–35.

83. *Shanghan zongbing lun*, 1.151–52.

84. The same claim that cold damage disorders did not exist in the south appears later in Vietnam, in the eighteenth century. For a recent discussion of this claim in Vietnamese history, see Leung, "'South' Imagined and Lived."

85. Extant records regarding Pang Anshi, such as his biography in *Song shi* (462.13520–22) and Su Shi's letters to him, pertain mainly to his activities in Hubei and Anhui and did not show that he had been to the far south in person.

86. *Junzhai dushuzhi jiaozheng*, 15.708.

87. *Lingnan weisheng fang, shang*, 6.

88. Leung notes the increasing importance of the northwest-southeast/north-south axes in Yuan, Ming, and Qing medicine and ascribes it to the long-term political division between the Southern Song and Jin governments. The analysis of "Ten Talks" here provides a more specific explanation of how this political division affected the increasingly prominent role of the north-south axis in medicine; that is, northern physicians' ineffective treatments of *zhang* disorders in Lingnan stimulated medical authors there to use the long-existing axis in medical writings to explain those physicians' failures. Leung, "Jibing yu fangtu zhi guanxi," 170–71.

89. *Guihai yuheng zhi*, 130.

90. *Lingnan weisheng fang, shang*, 22–23.

91. *Lingnan weisheng fang, shang,* 23.

92. *Lingnan weisheng fang, shang,* 23.

93. *Lingwai daida jiaozhu,* 4.152–53.

Conclusion

1. On the author and circulation of *Lüchan Rocks* and the location of Ciyun Mountain, see Zheng, "*Lü chanyan bencao* jiaozhu houji." On the boom of writings on West Lake, see Duan, *Rise of West Lake,* 79–104.

2. Wang Jie, *Lüchanyan bencao, shang,* 10.

3. *Hongshi jiyan fang kaozhu,* 4.57.

4. *Hongshi jiyan fang kaozhu,* 2.17.

5. For detailed analysis of information sources collected in *Mr. Hong's Collection of Effective Formulas,* see Qian Chaochen, "Hou ji," in *Hongshi jiyan fang kaozhu,* 93–105.

6. *Yeshi luyan fang,* postscript, 249.

7. *Weishi jiacang fang,* preface, 3.

8. *Yijian zhi,* 185.

9. *Baoqing bencao zhezhong,* 3.470.

10. The same priority of authoritative medical texts over empirical practices can also been seen in records of "breast abscesses" (*ruyong*) in imperial medical literature. See Chin, "Zhongguo chuantong yiji zhongde ruyong."

11. See, for example, *Renzhai zhizhi fanglun,* 25.316.

12. *Huoren shizheng fang houji,* table of contents (*mulu*), 507.

13. *Yijian fang jiumiu,* 1.253–57.

14. The Northern and Southern Song courts revised, expanded, renamed, and printed *The Imperial Pharmacy's Formulary* several times. On the bibliographic information that accompanied this formulary, see Goldschmidt, "Commercializing Medicine"; and Liu Shu-fen, "Tang Song shiqi sengren, guojia, han yiliao de guanxi."

15. Goldschmidt, "Commercializing Medicine," 344–45; Smith, *Forgotten Disease,* 76–84.

16. Leung, "Medical Instruction and Popularization"; Chao, *Medicine and Society.*

17. Grant, *Chinese Physician,* 55–60.

18. For analyses of the literary styles applied in *yi'an* books, see, for instance, Zeitlin, "Literary Fashioning"; and Kirk, "Rhetoric, Treatment and Authority."

19. To be sure, in addition to the *yi'an* genre, other medical subgenres in the Ming era also presented case narratives. See, for example, Chang, "Aishen nianzhong" and "Yiqie jiewang." Existing scholarship has not yet, however, reached consensus over the most salient features of the case narratives in those subgenres. To maintain a clear focus for this comparative analysis, I therefore do not discuss such cases in this study.

20. Furth, "Introduction," 3.

21. *Hanshi yitong, shang*, 2–3.

22. *Maiyu, xia*, 193.

23. *Hanshi yitong, shang*, 2–3.

24. *Weishi jiacang fang*, preface, 3.

25. Ye Linzhi, preface, in *Huoren shizheng fang*, 19.

26. Cullen, "*Yi'an* (Case Statements)," 314–16.

27. Cheng Lu, preface, in *Shishan yi'an*, 3.

28. *Maiyu, xia*, 193.

29. Cullen, "*Yi'an* (Case Statements)," 314–16; Furth, "Introduction," 5–13.

30. My understanding of the development of medical case narratives in premodern and early modern Europe draws heavily on Pomata, "Sharing Cases" and "Medical Case Narrative."

31. On interpersonal familiarity as the basis of trust in premodern England, see Shapin, *Social History of Truth*.

32. Leong and Rankin, "Testing Drugs."

33. Andrews, *Making of Modern Chinese Medicine*; Lei, *Neither Donkey nor Horse*.

34. Lei, "How Did Chinese Medicine Become Experiential?"

Bibliography

Primary Sources (Listed by Title)

Baoqing bencao zhezhong 寶慶本草折衷, by Chen Yan 陳衍 (13th century). In *Nan Song zhenxi bencao sanzhong* 南宋珍稀本草三種, edited by Zheng Jinsheng 鄭金生. Beijing: Renmin Weisheng Chubanshe, 2007.

Beihu lu 北戶錄, by Duan Gonglu 段公路 (fl. late 9th century). In *Zhongguo lishi dili wenxian jikan* 中國歷史地理文獻輯刊, vol. 35. Shanghai: Shanghai Jiaotong Daxue Chubanshe, 2009.

Beiji qianjin yaofang 備急千金要方, by Sun Simiao 孫思邈 (ca. 581–682). In *Qianjin fang* 千金方, edited by Liu Gengsheng 劉更生 and Zhang Ruixian 張瑞賢. Beijing: Huaxia Chubanshe, 1996.

Beimeng suoyan 北夢瑣言, by Sun Guangxian 孫光憲 (896–968). In *Quan Song biji* 全宋筆記, ser. 1, vol. 1. Zhengzhou: Daxiang Chubanshe, 2003.

Beishan jiujing 北山酒經, by Zhu Gong 朱肱 (1068–1165). In *Siku quanshu*, Wenyuange edition 文淵閣四庫全書, vol. 844. Taipei: Taiwan Shangwu Yinshuguan, 1983–86.

Bencao shiyi jishi 本草拾遺輯釋, by Chen Cangqi 陳藏器 (ca. 687–757). Edited by Shang Zhijun 尚志鈞. Hefei: Anhui Kexuejishu Chubanshe, 2002.

Bencao yanyi 本草衍義, by Kou Zongshi 寇宗奭 (fl. early 12th century). Beijing: Renmin Weisheng Chubanshe, 1990.

Bencaojing jizhu 本草經集注, by Tao Hongjing 陶弘景 (456–536). Edited by Shang Zhijun 尚志鈞 and Shang Yuansheng 尚元勝. Beijing: Renmin Weisheng Chubanshe, 1994.

Benshi shi 本事詩, by Meng Qi 孟棨 (9th century). In *Benshi shi, Xu benshi shi, Benshi ci* 本事詩、續本事詩、本事詞, edited by Li Xueying 李學穎. Shanghai: Shanghai Guji Chubanshe, 1991.

Boji fang 博濟方, by Wang Gun 王袞 (11th century). Edited by Wang Zhenguo 王振國 and Song Yongmei 宋詠梅. Shanghai: Shanghai Kexuejishu Chubanshe, 2003.

Daoxiang ji 道鄉集, by Zou Hao 鄒浩 (1060–1111). In *Siku quanshu*, Wenyuange edition 文淵閣四庫全書, vol. 1121. Taipei: Taiwan Shangwu Yinshuguan, 1983–86.

Er Cheng ji 二程集, by Cheng Hao 程顥 (1032–1085) and Cheng Yi 程頤 (1033–1107). Edited by Wang Xiaoyu 王孝魚. Beijing: Zhonghua Shuju, 2004.

Erya 爾雅. Edited by Zhou Yuanfu 周遠富 and Yu Ruo 愚若. Beijing: Zhonghua Shuju, 2020.

Erya shu 爾雅疏, edited by Xing Bing 邢昺 (932–1010). In *Shandong wenxian jicheng* 山東文獻集成, ser. 4, vol. 10. Jinan: Shandong Daxue Chubanshe, 2011.

Guihai yuheng zhi 桂海虞衡志, by Fan Chengda 范成大 (1126–1193). In *Fan Chengda biji liuzhong* 范成大筆記六種, edited by Kong Fanli 孔凡禮. Beijing: Zhonghua Shuju, 2002.

Han shu 漢書, by Ban Gu 班固 (32–92). Beijing: Zhonghua Shuju, 1962.

Hanshi yitong 韓氏醫通, by Han Mao 韓懋 (1441–1522?). In *Zhonghua yishu jicheng* 中華醫書集成, vol. 25. Beijing: Zhongyiguji Chubanshe, 1999.

Helin yulu 鶴林玉露, by Luo Dajing 羅大經 (1196–after 1252). In *Quan Song biji* 全宋筆記, ser. 8, vol. 3. Zhengzhou: Daxiang Chubanshe, 2017.

Hongshi jiyan fang kaozhu 洪氏集驗方考注, by Hong Zun 洪遵 (1120–174). Edited by Qian Chaochen 錢超塵. Beijing: Xueyuan Chubanshe, 2009.

Hou Han shu 後漢書, by Fan Ye 范曄 (398–445). Beijing: Zhonghua Shuju, 1965.

Huoren shizheng fang 活人事證方, by Liu Xinfu 劉信甫. In *Zhenban haiwaihuigui zhongyiguji congshu* 珍版海外回歸中醫古籍叢書, vol. 1. Beijing: Renmin Weisheng Chubanshe, 2008.

Huoren shizheng fang houji 活人事證方後集, by Liu Xinfu 劉信甫 (13th century). In *Zhenban haiwaihuigui zhongyiguji congshu* 珍版海外回歸中醫古籍叢書, vol. 1. Beijing: Renmin Weisheng Chubanshe, 2008.

Jianyan yilai xinian yaolu 建炎以來繫年要錄, by Li Xinchuan 李心傳 (1166–1243). Beijing: Zhonghua Shuju, 1956.

Jiu Tang shu 舊唐書, by Liu Xu 劉昫 (887–946) et al. Beijing: Zhonghua Shuju, 1975.

Junzhai dushuzhi jiaozheng 郡齋讀書志校證, by Chao Gongwu 晁公武 (1105–1180). Edited by Sun Meng 孫猛. Shanghai: Shanghai Guji Chubanshe, 2005.

Kaibao bencao (jifu ben) 開寶本草 (輯復本), by Lu Duoxun 盧多遜 (934–985) et al. Edited by Shang Zhijun 尚志鈞. Hefei: Anhui Kexuejishu Chubanshe, 1998.

Lingbiao luyi jiaobu 嶺表錄異校補, by Liu Xun 劉恂 (fl. late 9th century). Edited by Shang Bi 商璧 and Pan Bo 潘博. Nanning: Guangxi Minzu Chubanshe, 1988.

Lingnan weisheng fang 嶺南衛生方, compiled by Shi Jihong 釋繼洪 (13th century). Shanghai: Shanghai Keji Chubanshe, 2003.

Lingwai daida jiaozhu 嶺外代答校注, by Zhou Qufei 周去非 (1135–1189). Edited by Yang Wuquan 楊武泉. Beijing: Zhonghua Shuju, 1999.

Liu Yuxi quanji biannian jiaozhu 劉禹錫全集編年校注, by Liu Yuxi 劉禹錫

(772–842). Edited by Tao Min 陶敏 and Tao Hongyu 陶紅雨. Changsha: Yuelu Shushe, 2003.

Lou Yue ji 樓鑰集, by Lou Yue 樓鑰 (1137–1213). Edited by Gu Dapeng 顧大朋. Hangzhou: Zhejiang Guji Chubanshe, 2010.

Lüchanyan bencao 履巉岩本草, by Wang Jie 王介 (fl. early 13th century). In *Nan Song zhenxi bencao sanzhong* 南宋珍稀本草三種, edited by Zheng Jinsheng 鄭金生. Beijing: Renmin Weisheng Chubanshe, 2007.

Lüshe beiyao fang 旅舍備要方, by Dong Ji 董汲 (fl. 1102–1117). Shanghai: Shanghai Kexuejishu Chubanshe, 2003.

Maiyu 脈語, by Wu Kun 吳昆 (1552–?). In *Wu Kun yixue quanshu* 吳昆醫學全書, edited by Guo Junshuang 郭君雙. Beijing: Zhongguo Zhongyiyao Chubanshe, 1999.

Mingdao zazhi 明道雜誌, by Zhang Lei 張耒 (1054–1114). In *Quan Song biji* 全宋筆記, ser. 2, vol. 7. Zhengzhou: Daxiang Chubanshe, 2006.

Nan shi 南史, by Li Yanshou 李延壽 (fl. 7th century). Beijing: Zhonghua Shuju, 1975.

Nanyang huoren shu 南陽活人書 (*Shanghan baiwen* 傷寒百問), by Zhu Gong 朱肱 (1068–1165). In *Zhu Gong, Pang Anshi yixue quanshu* 朱肱、龐安時醫學全書, edited by Tian Sisheng 田思勝. Beijing: Zhongguo Zhongyiyao Chubanshe, 2006.

Puji benshifang 普濟本事方, by Xu Shuwei 許叔微 (1079–1154). In *Xu Shuwei yixue quanshu* 許叔微醫學全書, edited by Liu Jingchao 劉景超 and Li Jushuang 李具雙. Beijing: Zhongguo Zhongyiyao Chubanshe, 2006.

Quan Song wen 全宋文, compiled by Zeng Zaozhuang 曾棗莊 and Liu Lin 劉琳. Chengdu: Bashu Shushe, 1988–94.

Renzhai zhizhi fanglun 仁齋直指方論, by Yang Shiying 楊士瀛 (13th century). In *Yang Shiying yixue quanshu* 楊士瀛醫學全書, edited by Lin Huiguang 林慧光. Beijing: Zhongguo Zhongyiyao Chubanshe, 2006.

Shanghan baizheng ge 傷寒百證歌, by Xu Shuwei 許叔微. A manuscript facsimile of a printed Yuan-dynasty edition, in the National Central Library, Taiwan.

Shanghan jiushi lun 傷寒九十論. Authorship is under debate. In *Xu Shuwei yixue quanshu* 許叔微醫學全書, edited by Liu Jingchao 劉景超 and Li Jushuang 李具雙. Beijing: Zhongguo Zhongyiyao Chubanshe, 2006.

Shanghan lun 傷寒論 (*Shanghan zabing lun* 傷寒雜病論), by Zhang Ji 張機 (150–219). In *Song ben "Shanghan lun" wenxian shilun* 宋本《傷寒論》文獻史論, edited by Qian Chaochen 錢超塵. Beijing: Xueyuan Chubanshe, 2015.

Shanghan zongbing lun 傷寒總病論, by Pang Anshi 龐安時 (ca. 1043–1100). In *Zhu Gong, Pang Anshi yixue quanshu* 朱肱、龐安時醫學全書, edited by Tian Sisheng 田思勝. Beijing: Zhongguo Zhongyiyao Chubanshe, 2006.

Shen Kuo quanji 沈括全集, by Shen Kuo 沈括 (1031–1095). Edited by Yang Weisheng 楊渭生. Hangzhou: Zhejiang Daxue Chubanshe, 2011.

Shi Zaizhi fang 史載之方, by Shi Kan 史堪 (fl. early 12th century). Shanghai: Shanghai Kexuejishu Chubanshe, 2003.

Shiji 史記, by Sima Qian 司馬遷 (ca. 145 BCE–?). Beijing: Zhonghua Shuju, 2014.

Shishan yi'an 石山醫案, by Wang Ji 汪機 (1463–1539). In *Ming Qing shibajia mingyi yi'an* 明清十八家名醫醫案, edited by Yi Guangqian 伊廣謙 and Li Zhanyong 李占永. Beijing: Zhongguo Zhongyiyao Chubanshe, 1996.

Sima Guang ji 司馬光集, by Sima Guang 司馬光 (1019–1086). Edited by Li Wenze 李文澤 and Xia Shaohui 霞紹暉. Chengdu: Sichuan Daxue Chubanshe, 2010.

Song da zhaoling ji 宋大詔令集, edited by Song Shou 宋綬 (991–1040) and Song Minqiu 宋敏求. Beijing: Zhonghua Shuju, 1962.

Song huiyao jigao 宋會要輯稿, compiled by Xu Song 徐松 (1781–1848). Edited by Liu Lin 劉麟, Dioa Zhongmin 刁忠民, Shu Dagang 舒大剛, and Yin Bo 尹波. Shanghai: Shanghai Guji Chubanshe, 2014.

Song shi 宋史, by Tuotuo (Toktoghan) 脫脫 (1314–1355) et al. Beijing: Zhonghua Shuju, 1977.

Su Shen neihan liangfang 蘇沈內翰良方, by Su Shi 蘇軾 (1037–1101) and Shen Kuo 沈括. In *Shen Kuo quanji* 沈括全集, vol. 3.

Su Shi wenji 蘇軾文集, by Su Shi 蘇軾. Edited by Kong Fanli 孔凡禮. Beijing: Zhonghua Shuju, 1986.

Su weigong wenji 蘇魏公文集, by Su Song 蘇頌 (1020–1101). Edited by Wang Tongce 王同策, Guan Chengxue 管成學, and Yan Zhongqi 顔中其. Beijing: Zhonghua Shuju, 1988.

Sui shu 隋書, by Wei Zheng 魏徵 (580–643) et al. Beijing: Zhonghua Shuju, 1973.

Suichutang shumu 遂初堂書目, by You Mao 尤袤 (1127–1194). In *Song Yuan Ming Qing shumu tiba congkan* 宋元明清書目題跋叢刊, vol. 1. Beijing: Zhonghua Shuju, 2006.

Taiping guangji 太平廣記, compiled by Li Fang 李昉 (925–996) et al. Beijing: Zhonghua Shuju, 1995.

Taiping shenghui fang 太平聖惠方, by Wang Huaiyin 王懷隱 (925–997) et al. Beijing: Renmin Weisheng Chubanshe, 1958.

Waitai miyao fang 外臺秘要方, by Wang Tao 王燾 (670–755). Edited by Gao Wenzhu 高文鑄. Beijing: Huaxia Chubanshe, 1997.

Weishi jiacang fang 魏氏家藏方, by Wei Xian 魏峴 (ca. 1192–?). In *Haiwaihuigui zhongyi shanbenguji congshu (xu)* 海外回歸中醫善本古籍叢書 (續), vol. 5. Beijing: Renmin Weisheng Chubanshe, 2010.

Xiaoer yaozheng zhijue 小兒藥證直訣, compiled by Yan Jizhong 閻季忠 (fl. early 12th century). In *Qian Yi, Liu Fang yixue quanshu* 錢乙、劉昉醫學全書, edited by Li Zhiyong 李志庸. Beijing: Zhongguo Zhongyiyao Chubanshe, 2005.

Xinbian furen daquan liangfang 新編婦人大全良方, by Chen Ziming 陳自明

(1190–1272). In *Zhonghua zaizao shanben* 中華再造善本. Beijing: Beijing Tushuguan Chubanshe, 2005.

Xinjiaozheng mengxi bitan 新校正夢溪筆談, by Shen Kuo 沈括. Edited by Hu Daojing 胡道靜. Hong Kong: Zhonghua Shuju, 1987.

Xu zizhi tongjian changbian 續資治通鑑長編, by Li Tao 李燾 (1115–1184). Beijing: Zhonghua Shuju, 1995.

Xuxiu Siku quanshu shanghan lei yizhu jicheng 續修四庫全書傷寒類醫著集成, vol. 1, edited by Yu Shun 虞舜, Wang Xuguang 王旭光, and Zhang Yucai 張玉才. Nanjing: Jiangsu Kexuejishu Chubanshe, 2010.

Yan fanlu xuji 演繁露續集, by Cheng Dachang 程大昌 (1123–1195). In *Quan Song biji* 全宋筆記, ser. 4, vol. 9. Zhengzhou: Daxiang Chubanshe, 2008.

Yeshi luyan fang 葉氏錄驗方, by Ye Dalian 葉大廉 (fl. late 12th century). Shanghai: Shanghai Kexuejishu Chubanshe, 2003.

Yifang leiju 醫方類聚, compiled by Kim Ye-mong 金禮蒙 (15th century) et al. Beijing: Renmin Weisheng Chubanshe, 1981–82.

Yijian fang jiumiu 易簡方糾謬, by Lu Tan 盧檀 (13th century). In *Yongjia yipai yanjiu* 永嘉醫派研究, by Liu Shijue 劉時覺. Beijing: Zhongyiguji Chubanshe, 2000.

Yijian zhi 夷堅志, by Hong Mai 洪邁 (1123–1202). Edited by He Zhuo 何卓. Beijing: Zhonghua Shuju, 1981.

Yijing zhengbenshu 醫經正本書, by Cheng Jiong 程迥 (fl. late 12th century). In *Zhuzi jicheng xubian* 諸子集成續編, vol. 12. Chengdu: Sichuan Renmin Chubanshe, 1998.

Yingguo Aboding daxue tushuguancang "Yongle dadian" 英國阿伯丁大學圖書館藏《永樂大典》, by Xie Jin 解縉 (1369–1415) et al. Beijing: Guojiatushu Chubanshe, 2016.

Yishuo 醫説, by Zhang Gao 張杲 (1149–1227). In *Zhonghua zaizao shanben* 中華再造善本. Beijing: Beijing Tushuguan Chubanshe, 2006.

Yongle dadian 永樂大典, by Xie Jin 解縉 et al. Beijing: Zhonghua Shuju, 1986.

Youyang zazu jiaojian 酉陽雜組校箋, by Duan Chengshi 段成式 (803?–863). Edited by Xu Yiming 許逸明. Beijing: Zhonghua Shuju, 2015.

Yuexi wenzai 粵西文載, compiled by Wang Sen 汪森 (1653–1726). In *Siku quanshu*, Wenyuange edition 文淵閣四庫全書, vol. 1465. Taipei: Taiwan Shangwu Yinshuguan, 1983–86.

Yungu zaji 雲谷雜記, by Zhang Hao 張淏 (fl. late 12th century). In *Quan Song biji* 全宋筆記, ser. 7, vol. 1. Zhengzhou: Daxiang Chubanshe, 2015.

Yunzhuang ji 雲莊集, by Zeng Xie 曾協 (?–1173). Edited by Yu Shaohai 于少海. Nanchang: Jiangxi Jiaoyu Chubanshe, 2004.

Zengguang taiping huimin hejiju fang 增廣太平惠民和劑局方, by Chen Shiwen 陳師文 (fl. early 12th century) et al. Haikou: Hainan Chubanshe, 2002.

Zhizhai shulu jieti 直齋書錄解題, by Chen Zhensun 陳振孫 (1179–1262). Edited by

Xu Xiaoman 徐小蠻 and Gu Meihua 顧美華. Shanghai: Shanghai Guji Chubanshe, 1987.

Zhouhou beijifang 肘後備急方, by Ge Hong 葛洪 (283–343). Beijing: Renmin Weisheng Chubanshe, 1963.

Zhubing yuanhou lun jiaozhu 諸病源候論校注, by Chao Yuanfang 巢元方 (fl. early 7th century) et al. Edited by Ding Guangdi 丁光迪. Beijing: Renmin Weisheng Chubanshe, 1991.

Secondary Sources (Listed by author)

Allen, Sarah M. *Shifting Stories: History, Gossip, and Lore in Narratives from Tang Dynasty China*. Cambridge, MA: Harvard University Press, 2014.

Andrews, Bridie. "From Case Records to Case Histories: The Modernisation of a Chinese Medical Genre, 1912–49." In *Innovation in Chinese Medicine*, edited by Elisabeth Hsu, 324–36. Cambridge: Cambridge University Press, 2001.

———. *The Making of Modern Chinese Medicine, 1850–1960*. Vancouver: University of British Columbia Press, 2014.

Aoyama Sadao 青山定雄. *Tō Sō jidai no kōtsū to chishi chizu no kenkyū* 唐宋時代の交通と地誌地圖の研究. Tōkyō: Yoshikawa Kōbunkan, 1969.

Beijing Tushuguan 北京圖書館, ed. *Zhongguo banke tulu* 中國版刻圖錄. Beijing: Wenwu Chubanshe, 1961.

Bian, He. "Documenting Medications: Patients' Demand, Physicians' Virtuosity, and Genre-Mixing of Prescription-Cases (*Fang'an*) in Seventeenth-Century China." *Early Science and Medicine* 22, no. 1 (March 2017): 103–23.

———. "An Ever-Expanding Pharmacy: Zhao Xuemin and the Conditions for New Knowledge in Eighteenth-Century China." *Harvard Journal of Asiatic Studies* 77, no. 2 (December 2017): 287–319.

———. *Know Your Remedies: Pharmacy and Culture in Early Modern China*. Princeton, NJ: Princeton University Press, 2020.

Bol, Peter K. "A Literati Miscellany and Sung Intellectual History: The Case of Chang Lei's *Ming-Tao Tsa-Chih*." *Journal of Sung-Yuan Studies* 25 (1995): 121–51.

———. *Neo-Confucianism in History*. Cambridge, MA: Harvard University Asia Center, 2008.

———. "Reconceptualizing the Order of Things in Northern and Southern Song." In *The Cambridge History of China, Vol. 5, Pt. 2: Sung China, 960–1279*, edited by John W. Chaffee and Denis Twitchett, 665–726. Cambridge: Cambridge University Press, 2015.

———. *This Culture of Ours: Intellectual Transitions in T'ang and Sung China*. Stanford, CA: Stanford University Press, 1992.

Bossler, Beverly. *Powerful Relations: Kinship, Status, and the State in Sung China (960–1279)*. Cambridge, MA: Harvard University Press, 1998.

Boyanton, Stephen. "The Hermeneutics of a Song Dynasty Case Record." Asian Medicine Zone (curated website), November 25, 2015, www.asianmedicinezone.com/chinese-east-asian/hermeneutics-song-dynasty-case-record.

———. "The *Treatise on Cold Damage* and the Formation of Literati Medicine: Social, Epidemiological, and Medical Change in China, 1000–1400." PhD diss., Columbia University, 2015.

Bretelle-Establet, Florence. "The Worst Environment in Which to Live in China: A Question of Points of View. The Legendary Miasmatic Far South of China Challenged by Local Doctors in Late Imperial China." In *Making Sense of Health, Disease, and the Environment in Cross-Cultural History: The Arabic-Islamic World, China, Europe, and North America*, edited by Florence Bretelle-Establet, Marie Gaille, and Mehrnaz Katouzian-Safadi, 165–208. Cham: Springer, 2019.

Brokaw, Cynthia. "On the History of the Book in China." In *Printing and Book Culture in Late Imperial China*, edited by Cynthia Brokaw and Kaiwing Chow, 3–54. Berkeley: University of California Press, 2005.

Brown, Miranda. *The Art of Medicine in Early China: The Ancient and Medieval Origins of a Modern Archive*. New York: Cambridge University Press, 2015.

Burke, Peter. *What Is the History of Knowledge?* Cambridge: Polity Press, 2016.

Chaffee, John W. *The Thorny Gates of Learning in Sung China: A Social History of Examinations*. Cambridge: Cambridge University Press, 1985.

Chang Chia-feng 張嘉鳳. "Aishen nianzhong: *Zhegong manlu* (1635) zhong wenren zhi ji yu yang" 愛身念重——《折肱漫錄》(1635) 中文人之疾與養. *Taida lishixuebao* 臺大歷史學報 51 (June 2013): 1–80.

———. "Yiqie jiewang: *Zhegong manlu* de yangsheng yu zhishijiangou" 一切皆忘——《折肱漫錄》的養生與知識建構. In *Faguo hanxue* 法國漢學, vol. 18, edited by *Faguo hanxue* Congshu Bianji Weiyuanhui 《法國漢學》叢書編輯委員會, 187–210. Beijing: Zhonghua Shuju, 2019.

Chao, Yüan-ling. *Medicine and Society in Late Imperial China: A Study of Physicians in Suzhou, 1600–1850*. New York: Peter Lang, 2009.

Chen Hao 陳昊. *Ji zhi cheng shang—Qin-Song zhijian de jibing mingyi yu lishi xushi zhongde cunzai* 疾之成殤——秦宋之間的疾病名義與歷史敘事中的存在. Shanghai: Shanghai Guji Chubanshe, 2020.

———. *Shenfen xushi yu zhishi biaoshu zhijian de yizhe zhiyi: 6–8 shiji Zhongguo de shuji zhixu, weiyizhiti, yu yixue shenfen de fuxian* 身分敘事與知識表述之間的醫者之意：6–8 世紀中國的書籍秩序、為醫之體與醫學身分的浮現. Shanghai: Shanghai Guji Chubanshe, 2019.

———. "Zai xieben yu yinben zhijian de fangshu: Songdai *Qianjin fang* de shujishi" 在

BIBLIOGRAPHY *187*

寫本與印本之間的方書——宋代《千金方》的書籍史. *Zhongyiyao zazhi* 中醫藥雜誌 24, no. 1 (December 2013): 69–85.

Chen Hsiu-fen 陳秀芬. "Shiwu, yaoshu, yu gudu: Song Yuan Ming 'tiaosheng' xingxiang de liubian" 食物、妖術與蠱毒——宋元明「挑生」形象的流變. *Hanxue yanjiu* 漢學研究 34, no. 3 (September 2016): 9–51.

Chen, Ruth Yun-ju 陳韻如. "The Quest for Efficiency: Knowledge Management in Medical Formularies." *Harvard Journal of Asiatic Studies* 80, no. 2 (December 2020): 347–80.

———. "Songdai shidafu canyu difang yishu kanyin xintan" 宋代士大夫參與地方醫書刊印新探. *Zhongyang yanjiuyuan lishi yuyan yanjiusuo jikan* 中央研究院歷史語言研究所集刊 92, no. 3 (September 2021): 437–507.

Chen Xiaolan 陳曉蘭. "*Xinbian leiyao tuzhu bencao* ji qi chuankeben kaocha" 《新編類要圖注本草》及其傳刻本考察. *Banben muluxue yanjiu* 版本目錄學研究 3 (January 2012): 231–44.

Chen Yuan-peng 陳元朋. "*Bencaojing jizhu* suozai 'Tao zhu' zhongde zhishi leixing, yaochan fenbu, yu beifang yaowu de shuru" 《本草經集注》所載"陶注"中的知識類型、藥產分布與北方藥物的輸入." *Zhongguo shehui lishi pinglun* 中國社會歷史評論 12 (June 2011): 184–212.

———. *Liang Song de "shangyi shiren" yu "ruyi": jianlun qi zai Jin-Yuan de liubian* 兩宋的「尚醫士人」與「儒醫」——兼論其在金元的流變. Taipei: Guoli Taiwan Daxue Chuban Weiyuanhui, 1997.

———. "Songdai ruyi" 宋代儒醫. In *Zhongguoshi xinlun: Yiliaoshi fence* 中國史新論: 醫療史分冊, edited by Shengming Yiliaoshi Yanjiushi 生命醫療史研究室, 245–305. Taipei: Lianjing Chuban Shiye Gongsi, 2015.

———. "Zhongyaocai niuhuang de shengchan lishi ji qi bencaoyaotu suo sheji de zhishijiegou" 中藥材牛黃的生產歷史及其本草藥圖所涉及的知識結構. *Gugong xueshu jikan* 故宮學術季刊 36, no. 4 (December 2019): 35–60.

Cheng, Hsiao-wen. *Divine, Demonic, and Disordered: Women without Men in Song Dynasty China*. Seattle: University of Washington Press, 2021.

Cherniack, Susan. "Book Culture and Textual Transmission in Sung China." *Harvard Journal of Asiatic Studies* 54, no. 1 (June 1994): 5–125.

Chia, Lucille. *Printing for Profit: The Commercial Publishers of Jianyang, Fujian (11th–17th Centuries)*. Cambridge, MA: Harvard University Asia Center for Harvard-Yenching Institute, 2002.

Chia, Lucille, and Hilde De Weerdt, eds. *Knowledge and Text Production in an Age of Print: China, 900–1400*. Leiden: Brill, 2011.

Chin Shih-chi 金仕起. "Chutu gudai yiliao xiangguan wenben de shuxie yu bianci" 出土古代醫療相關文本的書寫與編次. *Guoli zhengzhi daxue lishixuebao* 國立政治大學歷史學報 55 (May 2021): 1–84.

———. "Zhongguo chuantong yiji zhongde ruyong, xingbie, yu jingyan" 中國傳統醫籍中的乳癰、性別與經驗. *Guoli zhengzhi daxue lishixuebao* 國立政治大學歷史學報 47 (May 2017): 1–74.

———. *Zhongguo gudai de yixue, yishi, yu zhengzhi: yi yishi wenben wei zhongxin de yige fenxi* 中國古代的醫學、醫史與政治: 以醫史文本為中心的一個分析. Taipei: Zhengzhi Daxue Chubanshe, 2010.

Chittick, Andrew. "The Development of Local Writing in Early Medieval China." *Early Medieval China* 9 (2003): 35–70.

Chu Pingyi 祝平一. "Song-Ming zhiji de yishi yu 'ruyi'" 宋、明之際的醫史與「儒醫」. *Zhongyang yanjiuyuan lishi yuyan yanjiusuo jikan* 中央研究院歷史語言研究所集刊 77, no. 3 (September 2006): 401–48.

Crisciani, Chiara. "Histories, Stories, Exempla, and Anecdotes: Michele Savonarola from Latin to Vernacular." In *Historia: Empiricism and Erudition in Early Modern Europe*, edited by Gianna Pomata and Nancy G. Siraisi, 297–324. Cambridge, MA: MIT Press, 2005.

Cullen, Christopher. "*Yi'an* 醫案 (Case Statements): The Origins of a Genre of Chinese Medical Literature." In *Innovation in Chinese Medicine*, edited by Elisabeth Hsu, 297–323. Cambridge: Cambridge University Press, 2001.

De Pee, Christian. "Notebooks (*Biji*) and Shifting Boundaries of Knowledge in Eleventh-Century China." *Medieval Globe* 3, no. 1 (2017): 129–67.

De Weerdt, Hilde. *Information, Territory, and Networks: The Crisis and Maintenance of Empire in Song China*. Cambridge, MA: Harvard University Press, 2016.

Dean-Jones, Lesley. "*Autopsia, Historia*, and What Women Know: The Authority of Women in Hippocratic Gynaecology." In *Knowledge and the Scholarly Medical Traditions*, edited by Don Bates, 41–59. Cambridge: Cambridge University Press, 1995.

Deng Xiaonan 鄧小南. *Songdai wenguan xuanren zhidu zhucengmian (xiuding ben)* 宋代文官選任制度諸層面 (修訂本). Beijing: Zhonghua Shuju, 2021.

Despeux, Catherine. "The System of the Five Circulatory Phases and the Six Seasonal Influences (*wuyun liuqi*), a Source of Innovation in Medicine under the Song (960–1279)." In *Innovation in Chinese Medicine*, edited by Elisabeth Hsu, 121–65. Cambridge: Cambridge University Press, 2001.

Duan, Xiaolin. *The Rise of West Lake: A Cultural Landmark in the Song Dynasty*. Seattle: University of Washington Press, 2020.

Ebrey, Patricia B. *Emperor Huizong*. Cambridge, MA: Harvard University Press, 2014.

Ebrey, Patricia B., and Maggie Bickford, eds. *Emperor Huizong and Late Northern Song China: The Politics of Culture and the Culture of Politics*. Cambridge, MA: Harvard University Press, 2006.

Ebrey, Patricia B., and Shih-shan Susan Huang, eds. *Visual and Material Cultures in Middle Period China*. Leiden: Brill, 2017.

Egan, Ronald. *The Problem of Beauty: Aesthetic Thought and Pursuits in Northern Song Dynasty China*. Cambridge, MA: Harvard University Asia Center, 2006.

——. "Shen Kuo Chats with Ink Stone and Writing Brush." In *Idle Talk: Gossip and Anecdote in Traditional China*, edited by Jack W. Chen and David Schaberg, 132–53. Berkeley: Global, Area, and International Archive, University of California Press, 2014.

——. "To Count Grains of Sand on the Ocean Floor: Changing Perceptions of Books and Learning in the Song Dynasty." In *Knowledge and Text Production in an Age of Print*, 33–62. Leiden: Brill, 2011.

Elman, Benjamin A. *On Their Own Terms: Science in China, 1550–1900*. Cambridge, MA: Harvard University Press, 2005.

Fan Ka Wai 范家偉. *Bei Song jiaozheng yishuju xintan: Yi guojia yu yixue wei zhongxin* 北宋校正醫書局新探: 以國家與醫學為中心. Hong Kong: Zhonghua Shuju, 2014.

——. *Dayi jingcheng: Tangdai guojia xinyang yu yixue* 大醫精誠: 唐代國家、信仰與醫學. Taipei: Dongda Tushu Chubanshe, 2007.

——. "*Ge Xianweng zhouhou beijifang*" 葛仙翁肘後備急方. In *Early Medieval Chinese Texts: A Bibliographical Guide*, edited by Cynthia L. Chennault, Keith N. Knapp, Alan J. Berkowitz, and Albert E. Dien, 88–94. Berkeley: Institute of East Asian Studies, 2015.

——. *Liuchao Sui Tang yixue zhi chuancheng yu zhenghe* 六朝隋唐醫學之傳承與整合. Hong Kong: Zhongwen Daxue Chubanshe, 2004.

——. "Songdai yixue fazhan de waiyuan yinsu: ping Guo Zhisong *Zhongyiyao de yanbian: Songdai (960–1200)*" 宋代醫學發展的外緣因素--評郭志松 《中醫藥的演變: 宋代 (960–1200 年)》. *Zhongguo kejishi zazhi* 中國科技史雜志 31, no. 3 (September 2010): 328–36.

——. "Weijinnanbeichao Sui Tang shiqi de yixue" 魏晉南北朝隋唐時期的醫學. In *Zhongguoshi xinlun: Yiliaoshi fence*, edited by Shengming Yiliaoshi Yanjiushi 生命醫療史研究室, 151–93. Taipei: Lianjing Chuban Shiye Gongsi, 2015.

——. *Zhonggu shiqi de yizhe yu bingzhe* 中古時期的醫者與病者. Shanghai: Fudan Daxue Chubanshe, 2010.

Fang Chengfeng 方誠峰. "Yubi, yubi shouzhao, yu Bei Song Huizong chao de tongzhi fangshi" 御筆、御筆手詔與北宋徽宗朝的統治方式. *Hanxue yanjiu* 漢學研究 31, no. 3 (September 2013): 31–67.

Fang Rui 房銳. *Sun Guangxian yu "Beimeng suoyan" yanjiu* 孫光憲與 《北夢瑣言》研究. Beijing: Zhonghua Shuju, 2006.

Feng, H. Y., and J. K. Shryock. "The Black Magic in China Known as *Ku*." *Journal of the American Oriental Society* 55, no. 1 (March 1935): 1–30.

Feng Hanyong 馮漢鏞. *Gu fangshu jiyi* 古方書輯佚. Beijing: Renmin Weisheng Chubanshe, 1993.

Fried, Daniel. "Song Dynasty Classicism and the Eleventh Century 'Print Modernity.'" In *Comparative Print Culture: A Study of Alternative Literary Modernities*, edited by Rasoul Aliakbari, 23–39. London: Palgrave Macmillan, 2020.

Fu, Daiwie. "A Contextual and Taxonomic Study of the 'Divine Marvels' and 'Strange Occurrences' in the *Mengxi Bitan*." *East Asian Science, Technology, and Medicine* 11, no. 1 (1993–94): 3–35.

———. "The Flourishing of *Biji* or Pen-Notes Texts and Its Relations to History of Knowledge in Song China (960–1279)." *Extrême-Orient, Extrême-Occident*, hors série 29 (2007): 103–30.

Furth, Charlotte. "Introduction: Thinking with Cases." In *Thinking with Cases: Specialist Knowledge in Chinese Cultural History*, edited by Charlotte Furth, Judith Zeitlin, and Ping-chen Hsiung, 1–28. Honolulu: University of Hawai'i Press, 2007.

———. "The Physician as Philosopher of the Way: Zhu Zhenheng (1282–1358)." *Harvard Journal of Asiatic Studies* 66, no. 2 (December 2006): 423–59.

———. "Producing Medical Knowledge through Cases: History, Evidence, and Action." In *Thinking with Cases: Specialist Knowledge in Chinese Cultural History*, edited by Charlotte Furth, Judith Zeitlin, and Ping-chen Hsiung, 125–51.

Furth, Charlotte, Judith Zeitlin, and Ping-chen Hsiung, eds. *Thinking with Cases: Specialist Knowledge in Chinese Cultural History*. Honolulu: University of Hawai'i Press, 2007.

Genette, Gerard. *Paratexts: Thresholds of Interpretation*. Translated by Jane E. Lewin. New York: Cambridge University Press, 1997.

Goldschmidt, Asaf. "Commercializing Medicine or Benefiting the People—The First Public Pharmacy in China." *Science in Context* 21, no. 3 (October 2008): 311–50.

———. *The Evolution of Chinese Medicine: Song Dynasty, 960–1200*. London: Routledge, 2009.

———. "Huizong's Impact on Medicine and on Public Health." In *Emperor Huizong and Late Northern Song China: The Politics of Culture and the Culture of Politics*, edited by Patricia B. Ebrey and Maggie Bickford, 275–323. Cambridge, MA: Harvard University Press, 2006.

———. *Medical Practice in Twelfth-Century China—A Translation of Xu Shuwei's "Ninety Discussions [Cases] on Cold Damage Disorders."* Cham, Switzerland: Springer International Publishing: Imprint: Springer, 2019.

———. "Reasoning with Cases: The Transmission of Clinical Medical Knowledge in Twelfth-Century Song China." In *Antiquarianism, Language, and Medical Philology: From Early Modern to Modern Sino-Japanese Medical Discourses*, edited by Benjamin A. Elman, 19–51. Leiden: Brill, 2015.

Gong Shengsheng 龔勝生. "2000 nian lai Zhongguo zhang bing fenbu bianqian de chubu yanjiu" 2000年來中國瘴病分佈變遷的初步研究. *Dili xuebao* 地理學報 48, no. 4 (August 1993): 304–16.

Graham, Angus. *Two Chinese Philosophers: The Metaphysics of the Brothers Cheng*. La Salle, IL: Open Court, 1992.

Grant, Joanna. *A Chinese Physician: Wang Ji and the Stone Mountain Medical Case Histories*. London: Routledge, 2003.

Gu Hongyi 顧宏義. *Liang Song biji yanjiu* 兩宋筆記研究. Zhengzhou: Daxiang Chubanshe, 2020.

Han Yi 韓毅. *Songdai yixue fangshu de xingcheng yu chuanbo yingyong yanjiu* 宋代醫學方書的形成與傳播應用研究. Guangzhou: Guangdong Renmin Chubanshe, 2019.

Han Yi 韓毅 and Yu Boya 于博雅. "Nan Song Xu Shuwei yi'an yu linchuang jibing zhenliao chutan" 南宋許叔微醫案與臨床疾病診療初探. *Hebei daxue xuebao (zhexue shehuikexue ban)* 河北大學學報 (哲學社會科學版) 42, no. 6 (November 2017): 1–11.

Hanson, Marta. "From under the Elbow to Pointing to the Palm: Chinese Metaphors for Learning Medicine by the Book (Fourth–Fourteenth Centuries)." *BJHS Themes* 5 (2020): 75–92.

———. *Speaking of Epidemics in Chinese Medicine: Disease and the Geographic Imagination in Late Imperial China*. London: Routledge, 2011.

Hanson, Marta, and Gianna Pomata. "Medicinal Formulas and Experiential Knowledge in the Seventeenth-Century Epistemic Exchange between China and Europe." *Isis* 108, no. 1 (March 2017): 1–25.

Hargett, James M. "Historiography in Southern Sung Dynasty Local Gazetteers." In *The New and the Multiple: Sung Senses of the Past*, edited by Thomas H. C. Lee, 287–306. Hong Kong: Chinese University Press, 2004.

———. *Jade Mountains and Cinnabar Pools: The History of Travel Literature in Imperial China*. Seattle: University of Washington Press, 2018.

———. "Sketches." In *The Columbia History of Chinese Literature*, edited by Victor H. Mair, 560–65. New York: Columbia University Press, 2001.

———. "Song Dynasty Local Gazetteers and Their Place in the History of *Difangzhi* Writing." *Harvard Journal of Asiatic Studies* 56, no. 2 (December 1996): 405–42.

———. "The Travel Records (*Yu-chi*) of Su Shih (1037–1101)." *Hanxue yanjiu* 漢學研究 8, no. 2 (December 1990): 369–96.

———. *Treatises of the Supervisor and Guardian of the Cinnamon Sea: The Natural World and Material Culture of Twelfth-Century China*. Seattle: University of Washington Press, 2011.

———. "What Need Is There to Go Home? Travel as a Leisure Activity in the Travel

Records (*Youji* 游記) of Su Shi 蘇軾 (1037–1101)." *Chinese Historical Review* 23, no. 2 (2016): 111–29.

Harper, Donald. *Early Chinese Medical Literature: The Mawangdui Medical Manuscripts*. New York: Columbia University Press, 1998.

Hartman, Charles. *The Making of Song Dynasty History: Sources and Narratives, 960–1279 CE*. Cambridge: Cambridge University Press, 2021.

Hinrichs, TJ. "The Catchy Epidemic: Theorization and Its Limits in Han to Song Period Medicine." *East Asian Science, Technology, and Medicine* 41 (June 2015): 19–62.

———. "Governance through Medical Texts and the Role of Print." In *Knowledge and Text Production in an Age of Print: China*, 217–38. Leiden: Brill, 2011.

———. "The Medical Transforming of Governance and Southern Customs in Song Dynasty China (960–1279 CE)." PhD diss., Harvard University, 2003.

———. *Shamans, Witchcraft, and Quarantine of Governance and Southern Customs in Song China*. Unpublished manuscript.

———. "The Song and Jin Periods." In *Chinese Medicine and Healing: An Illustrated History*, edited by TJ Hinrichs and Linda Barnes, 97–127. Cambridge, MA: Belknap Press of Harvard University Press, 2013.

Hinrichs, TJ, and Linda L. Barnes, eds. *Chinese Medicine and Healing: An Illustrated History*. Cambridge, MA: Belknap Press of Harvard University Press, 2013.

Hofmann, Martin, Joachim Kurtz, and Ari Daniel Levine, eds. *Powerful Arguments: Standards of Validity in Late Imperial China*. Leiden; Boston: Brill, 2020.

Hong, Jeehee, and TJ Hinrichs. "Unwritten Life (and Death) of a 'Pharmacist' in Song China: Decoding Hancheng 韓城 Tomb Murals." *Cahiers d'Extrême-Asie* 24 (2015): 231–78.

Hsiao Fan 蕭璠. "Han Song jian wenxian suojian gudai Zhongguo nanfang de dili huanjing yu difangbing ji qi yingxiang" 漢宋間文獻所見古代中國南方的地理環境與地方病及其影響. *Zhongyang yanjiuyuan lishi yuyan yanjiusuo jikan* 中央研究院歷史語言研究所集刊 63, no. 1 (March 1993): 67–171.

Hsiung, Ping-chen. "Facts in the Tale: Case Records and Pediatric Medicine in Late Imperial China." In *Thinking with Cases: Specialist Knowledge in Chinese Cultural History*, edited by Charlotte Furth, Judith Zeitlin, and Ping-chen Hsiung, 152–68. Honolulu: University of Hawai'i Press, 2007.

Hsu, Elisabeth. *Pulse Diagnosis in Early Chinese Medicine: The Telling Touch*. Cambridge: Cambridge University Press, 2010.

Hu Daojing 胡道靜. "*Su Shen neihan liangfang* Chu Shu pan: Fenxi benshu meige fang lun suoshu de zuozhe: 'Shen fang' yiwei 'Su fang'" 《蘇沈內翰良方》楚蜀判—分析本書每個方、論所屬的作者: "沈方"抑為"蘇方." *Shehuikexue zhanxian* 社會科學戰線 3 (June 1980): 195–209.

Huang Jinming 黃瑾明 and Tang Nianguang 湯年光. "Guilin shike 'yangqi tang fang' kao" 桂林石刻「養氣湯方」考. *Guangxi zhongyiyao* 廣西中醫藥 2 (April 1980): 28–29.

Huang Kuan-chung 黃寬重. "Bei Song wanqi dui Guangxi de jinglüe: Yi Cheng Jie, Cheng Lin fuzi wei zhongxin de taolun" 北宋晚期對廣西的經略——以程節、程鄰父子為中心的討論. In *Faguo hanxue* 法國漢學, vol. 12, edited by *Faguo hanxue* Congshu Bianji Weiyuanhui 《法國漢學》叢書編輯委員會, 208–25. Beijing: Zhonghua Shuju, 2007.

———. *Nan Song shidai kang Jin de yijun* 南宋時代抗金的義軍. Taipei: Lianjing Chuban Shiye Gongsi, 1988.

Hymes, Robert P. "Gossip as History: Hong Mai's *Yijian zhi* and the Place of Oral Anecdotes in Song Historical Knowledge." *Chūgoku shigaku* 中国史学 21 (2011): 1–28.

———. "Not Quite Gentlemen? Doctors in Sung and Yuan." *Chinese Science* 8 (January 1987): 9–76.

———. *Statesmen and Gentlemen: The Elite of Fu-Chou, Chiang-Hsi, in Northern and Southern Sung*. Cambridge: Cambridge University Press, 1986.

Ihara Hiroshi 伊原弘. *Sōdai Chūgoku o tabisuru* 宋代中国を旅する. Tokyo: NTT Shuppan, 1995.

Inglis, Alister D. *Hong Mai's Record of the Listener and Its Song Dynasty Context*. Albany: State University of New York Press, 2006.

Jones, Claire. "Formula and Formulation: 'Efficacy Phrases' in Medieval English Medical Manuscripts." *Neuphilologische Mitteilungen* 99, no. 2 (1998): 199–209.

Keegan, David J. "The *Huang-ti nei-ching*: The Structure of the Compilation; the Significance of the Structure." PhD diss., University of California, Berkeley, 1988.

Kirk, Nalini. "Rhetoric, Treatment and Authority in the Medical Cases of Xiao Jing 蕭京 (1605–1672)." In *Thinking in Cases: Ancient Greek and Imperial Chinese Case Narratives*, edited by Markus Asper, 109–46. Berlin: De Gruyter, 2019.

Kurz, Johannes L. "The Politics of Collecting Knowledge: Song Taizong's Compilations Project." *T'oung pao* 通報 87, no. 4–5 (January 2001): 289–316.

Le Aiguo 樂愛國. *Zhuzi gewu zhizhilun yanjiu* 朱子格物致知論研究. Changsha: Yuelu Shushe, 2010.

Lee, Jen-der 李貞德. "Gender and Medicine in Tang China." *Asia Major* 16, no. 2 (2003): 1–32.

———. "Han Tang zhijian jiating zhongde jiankang zhaogu yu xingbie" 漢唐之間家庭中的健康照顧與性別. In *Disanjie guoji hanxue huiyi lunwenji: Xingbie yu yiliao* 第三屆國際漢學會議論文集: 性別與醫療, edited by Huang Ko-wu 黃克武, 1–49. Taipei: Zhongyang Yanjiuyuan Jindaishi Yanjiusuo, 2002.

———. "Han Tang zhijian yishu zhongde shengchan zhi dao" 漢唐之間醫書中的生產

之道. *Zhongyang yanjiuyuan lishi yuyan yanjiusuo jikan* 中央研究院歷史語言研究所集刊 67, no .3 (September 1996): 533–654.

———. "Juejing de lishi yanjiu: Cong 'gengnian qi' yici tanqi" 絕經的歷史研究——從「更年期」一詞談起. *Xin shixue* 新史學 29, no. 4 (December 2018): 179–223.

Lee, Thomas H. C. *Government Education and Examinations in Sung China*. Hong Kong: Chinese University Press, 1985.

Lei, Sean Hsiang-lin. "How Did Chinese Medicine Become Experiential? The Political Epistemology of *Jingyan*." *Positions: East Asia Cultures Critique* 10, no. 2 (2002): 333–64.

———. *Neither Donkey nor Horse: Medicine in the Struggle over China's Modernity*. Chicago: University of Chicago Press, 2014.

Leong, Elaine, and Alisha Rankin. "Testing Drugs and Trying Cures: Experiment and Medicine in Medieval and Early Modern Europe." *Bulletin of the History of Medicine* 91, no. 2 (Summer 2017): 157–82.

Leung, Angela Ki Che 梁其姿. "Jibing yu fangtu zhi guanxi: Yuan zhi Qing jian yijie de kanfa" 疾病與方土之關係: 元至清間醫界的看法. In *Disanjie guoji hanxue huiyi lunwenji: xingbie yu yiliao* 第三屆國際漢學會議論文集: 性別與醫療, 165–212. Taipei: Zhongyang Yanjiuyuan Jindaishi Yanjiusuo, 2002.

———. "Medical Instruction and Popularization in Ming-Qing China." *Late Imperial China* 24, no. 1 (June 2003): 130–52.

———. "Medical Learning from the Song to the Ming." In *The Song-Yuan-Ming Transition in Chinese History*, edited by Paul J. Smith and Richard von Glahn, 374–98. Cambridge, MA: Harvard University Asia Center, 2003.

———. "A 'South' Imagined and Lived: The Entanglement of Medical Things, Experts, and Identities in Premodern East Asia's South." In *Asia inside Out: Itinerant People*, edited by Eric Tagliacozzo, Helen F. Siu, and Peter C. Perdue, 122–45. Cambridge, MA: Harvard University Press, 2019.

Lewis, Mark Edward. *The Construction of Space in Early China*. Albany: State University of New York Press, 2005.

Li Jianmin 李建民. "Zhongguo gudai 'jinfang' kaolun" 中國古代「禁方」考論. *Zhongyang yanjiuyuan lishi yuyan yanjiusuo jikan* 中央研究院歷史語言研究所集刊 68, no. 1 (March 1997): 117–66.

Li Jingwei 李經緯. "Bei Song huangdi yu yixue" 北宋皇帝與醫學. *Zhongguo keji shiliao* 中國科技史料 10, no. 3 (June 1989): 3–20.

Li Shuhui 李淑慧. "*Su Shen liangfang* zuozhe qufen xinkao" 《蘇沈良方》作者區分新考. *Zhongyiwenxian zazhi* 中醫文獻雜誌 28, no. 3 (June 2010): 15–19.

———. "*Su Shen liangfang* zuozhe qufen xinkao (xuwan)" 《蘇沈良方》作者區分新考(續完). *Zhongyiwenxian zazhi* 中醫文獻雜誌 28, no. 4 (August 2010): 19–21.

Li Zhizhong 李致忠. "Yuan kan Xu Shuwei *Shanghan baizheng ge* yu *Shanghan fawei lun*" 元刊許叔微傷寒百證歌與傷寒發微論. *Shoucangjia* 收藏家 197 (March 2013): 41–46.

Liang Ken Yao 梁庚堯. "Cong nanbei dao dongxi: Songdai Zhenzhou zhuanyun diwei de zhuanbian" 從南北到東西——宋代真州轉運地位的轉變. *Taida lishixuebao* 臺大歷史學報 52 (November 2013): 53–143.

Lin Fu-shih 林富士. "'Jiusu' yu 'xinfeng': Shilun Songdai wuxi xinyang de tese" 「舊俗」與「新風」——試論宋代巫覡信仰的特色. *Xin shixue* 新史學 24, no. 4 (December 2013): 1–54.

Liu Ning 劉寧. "'Shihua' yu 'benshi': Zaitan *Liuyi shihua* yu wan Tang Wudai shige benshi zhuzuo de guanxi" 「詩話」與「本事」——再探《六一詩話》與晚唐五代詩歌本事著作的關係. *Tsinghua xuebao* 清華學報 48, no. 2 (June 2018): 327–56.

Liu Shu-fen 劉淑芬. "Tang Song shiqi sengren, guojia, han yiliao de guanxi: Cong yaofangdong dao huiminju" 唐、宋時期僧人、國家和醫療的關係: 從藥方洞到惠民局. In *Cong yiliao kan Zhongguoshi* 從醫療看中國史, edited by Li Jianmin 李建民, 145–202. Taipei: Lianjing Chuban Shiye Gongsi, 2008.

Liu, Yan. *Healing with Poisons: Potent Medicines in Medieval China.* Seattle: University of Washington Press, 2021.

Liu Yeqiu 劉葉秋. *Lidai biji gaishu* 歷代筆記概述. Beijing: Beijing Chubanshe, 2003.

Lloyd, Geoffrey, and Nathan Sivin. *The Way and the Word: Science and Medicine in Early China and Greece.* New Haven, CT: Yale University Press, 2002.

Lo, Vivienne. "The Han Period." In *Chinese Medicine and Healing: An Illustrated History*, edited by TJ Hinrichs and Linda Barnes, 31–64. Cambridge, MA: Belknap Press of Harvard University Press, 2013.

Lorge, Peter. *The Reunification of China: Peace through War under the Song Dynasty.* Cambridge: Cambridge University Press, 2015.

Lu Mingxin 逯銘昕. *Songdai shanghan xueshu yu wenxian kaolun* 宋代傷寒學術與文獻考論. Beijing: Kexue Chubanshe, 2016.

Ma Jixing 馬繼興. *Zhongyi wenxian xue* 中醫文獻學. Shanghai: Shanghai Kexuejishu Chubanshe, 1990.

Ma Lei 馬雷. "Lingnan, Wuling kao" 嶺南、五嶺考. *Zhonghua wenshi luncong* 中華文史論叢 120 (December 2015): 349–60, 400–401.

Mai, Huijun. "The Double Life of the Scallop: Anthropomorphic Biography, 'Pulu,' and the Northern Song Discourse on Things." *Journal of Song-Yuan Studies* 49 (2020): 149–205.

McDermott, Joseph P. *A Social History of the Chinese Book: Books and Literati Culture in Late Imperial China.* Hong Kong: Hong Kong University Press, 2006.

Métailié, Georges. "Lun Songdai bencao yu bowuxue zhuzuo zhongde lixue 'gewu' guan" 論宋代本草與博物學著作中的理學"格物"觀. Translated by Li Guoqiang

李國強. In *Faguo hanxue* 法國漢學, vol. 6, edited by Faguo hanxue Congshu Bianji Weiyuanhui 《法國漢學》叢書編輯委員會, 290–311. Beijing: Zhonghua Shuju, 2002.

———. *Science and Civilisation in China. Vol. 6, Biology and Biological Technology. Pt. 4, Traditional Botany: An Ethnobotanical Approach.* Translated by Janet Lloyd. Cambridge: Cambridge University Press, 2015.

Miyakawa Hisayuki 宮川尚志. "An Outline of the Naitō Hypothesis and Its Effects on Japanese Studies of China." *Far Eastern Quarterly* 14, no. 4 (August 1955): 533–52.

Miyashita Saburō 宮下三郎. "Malaria (*yao*) in Chinese Medicine during the Chin and Yüan Periods." *Acta Asiatica* 36 (September 1979): 90–112.

———. "Sō Gen no iryō" 宋元の医療. In *Sō Gen jidai no kagaku gijutsu shi* 宋元時代の科学技術史, edited by Kiyoshi Yabūchi 藪内清, 123–70. Kyōto: Kyōto Daigaku Jinbun Kagaku Kenkyūjo, 1967.

Okanishi Tameto 岡西為人. *Honzō gaisetsu* 本草概說. Osaka: Sōgensha, 1977.

———. *Song yiqian yiji kao* 宋以前醫籍考. Taipei: Nantian Shuju, 1977.

Peterson, Willard. "Another Look at Li 理." *Bulletin of Sung and Yüan Studies* 18 (1986): 13–31.

Pomata, Gianna. "The Medical Case Narrative: Distant Reading of an Epistemic Genre." *Literature and Medicine* 32, no. 1 (Spring 2014): 1–23.

———. "The Medical Case Narrative in Pre-Modern Europe and China: Comparative History of an Epistemic Genre." In *A Historical Approach to Casuistry: Norms and Exceptions in a Comparative Perspective*, edited by Carlo Ginzburg with Lucio Biasiori, 15–46. London: Bloomsbury, 2018.

———. "Observation Rising: Birth of an Epistemic Genre, 1500–1650." In *Histories of Scientific Observation*, edited by Lorraine Daston and Elizabeth Lunbeck, 45–80. Chicago: University of Chicago Press, 2011.

———. "Sharing Cases: The *Observationes* in Early Modern Medicine." *Early Science and Medicine* 15, no. 3 (2010): 193–236.

———. "A Word of the Empirics: The Ancient Concept of Observation and Its Recovery in Early Modern Medicine." *Annals of Science* 68, no. 1 (January 2011): 1–25.

Pomata, Gianna, and Nancy G. Siraisi. "Introduction." In *Historia: Empiricism and Erudition in Early Modern Europe*, edited by Gianna Pomata and Nancy G. Siraisi, 1–38. Cambridge, MA: MIT Press, 2005.

Qian Chaochen 錢超塵. "*Shanghan lun*" *wenxian tongkao* 傷寒論文獻通考. Beijing: Xueyuan Chubanshe, 1993.

———. "*Shanghan lun*" *wenxian xinkao* 《傷寒論》文獻新考. Beijing: Beijing Kexuejishu Chubanshe, 2018.

———. *Song ben "Shanghan lun" wenxian shilun* 宋本《傷寒論》文獻史論. Beijing: Xueyuan Chubanshe, 2015.

Reed, Carrie E. "Motivation and Meaning of a 'Hodge-Podge': Duan Chengshi's *Youyang Zazu*." *Journal of the American Oriental Society* 123, no. 1 (January–March 2003): 121–45.

Schafer, Edward H. *The Vermilion Bird: T'ang Images of the South*. Berkeley: University of California Press, 1967.

Shang, Zhijun 尚志鈞. "Tang Shenwei *Zhenglei bencao* yange" 唐慎微《證類本草》沿革. In *Zhenglei bencao: Chongxiu Zhenghe jingshi zhenglei beiyong bencao* 證類本草: 重修政和經史證類備用本草, edited by Shang Zhijun 尚志鈞, Zheng Jinsheng 鄭金生, Shang Yuanou 尚元藕, and Liu Dapei 劉大培, 3–5. Beijing: Huaxia Chubanshe, 1993.

Shapin, Steven. *A Social History of Truth: Civility and Science in Seventeenth-Century England*. Chicago: University of Chicago Press, 1994.

Shapin, Steven, and Simon Schaffer. *Leviathan and the Air-Pump: Hobbes, Boyle, and the Experimental Life*. Princeton, NJ: Princeton University Press, 2018.

Siebert, Martina. "Animals as Text: Producing and Consuming 'Text-Animals.'" In *Animals through Chinese History: Earliest Times to 1911*, edited by Roel Sterckx, Martina Siebert, and Dagmar Schäfer. Cambridge: Cambridge University Press, 2018.

———. "Consuming and Possessing Things on Paper: Examples from Late Imperial China's Natural Studies." In *Living the Good Life: Consumption in the Qing and Ottoman Empires of the Eighteenth Century*, edited by Elif Akçetin and Suraiya Faroqhi, 384–408. Leiden: Brill, 2018.

Sivin, Nathan. *Health Care in Eleventh-Century China*. New York: Springer, 2015.

———. "*Huang ti nei ching* 黃帝內經." In *Early Chinese Texts: A Bibliographical Guide*, edited by Michael Loewe, 196–215. Berkeley: Institute of East Asian Studies, University of California, Berkeley, 1993.

———. "A Seventh-Century Chinese Medical Case History." *Bulletin of the History of Medicine* 41, no. 3 (May–June 1967): 267–73.

———. "Shen Kua." In *Science in Ancient China: Researches and Reflections*, 1–53. Aldershot, UK: Variorum, 1995.

———. "Text and Experience in Classical Chinese Medicine." In *Knowledge and the Scholarly Medical Traditions*, edited by Don Bates, 177–204. Cambridge: Cambridge University Press, 1995.

Smith, Hilary. *Forgotten Disease: Illnesses Transformed in Chinese Medicine*. Stanford, CA: Stanford University Press, 2017.

Stanley-Baker, Michael. "JY146 *Ge xianweng zhouhou beijifang*" JY146 葛仙翁肘後備急方, translated by Huang Ruoze 黃若澤. In *Daozang jiyao.tiyao* 道藏輯要.提要, vol. 2, edited by Lai Chi Tim 黎志添, 809–19. Hong Kong: Xianggang Zhongwen Daxue Chubanshe, 2021.

Strickmann, Michel. "On the Alchemy of T'ao Hung-ching." In *Facets of Taoism: Essays* in *Chinese Religion*, edited by Holmes Welch and Anna Seidel, 123–92. New Haven, CT: Yale University Press, 1979.

Suzuki Masahiro鈴木正弘. "Dan Kōro sen *Hokutoroku* ni tsuite: Tō makki no rēnan ni kansuru hakubutsugaku teki chojutsu" 段公路撰《北戶錄》について——唐末期の嶺南に関する博物学的著述. *Risshō shigaku* 立正史学 79 (1996): 15–30.

Tian, Xiaofei. *Beacon Fire and Shooting Star: The Literary Culture of the Liang (502–57).* Cambridge, MA: Harvard University Press, 2007.

Tokunaga Yōsuke 德永洋介. "Sōdai no gyohitsu shushō" 宋代の御筆手詔. *Tōyōshi Kenkyū* 東洋史研究 57, no. 3 (December 1998): 393–426.

Tung, Yung-chang. "Confronting the Job Shortage: The Commercialization of Personnel Information in Song China." *Journal of Song-Yuan Studies* 48 (2019): 57–98.

Unschuld, Paul U. *Huang di nei jing Suwen: Nature, Knowledge, Imagery in an Ancient Chinese Medical Text.* Berkeley: University of California Press, 2003.

———. *Medicine in China: A History of Ideas.* Berkeley: University of California Press, 2010.

———. *Medicine in China: A History of Pharmaceutics.* Berkeley: University of California Press, 1986.

Wang Chengwen 王承文. "Tangdai Fang Qianli ji qi *Touhuang zalu* kaozheng" 唐代房千里及其《投荒雜錄》考證. In *Disanjie Zhong Ri xuezhe Zhongguo gudaishi luntan wenji* 第三屆中日學者中國古代史論壇文集, edited by Zhongguo Shehuikexue Yuan Lishi Yanjiusuo 中國社會科學院歷史研究所, Nippon Tōhō Gakkai 日本東方學會, and Wuhan Daxue San Zhi Jiu Shiji Yanjiusuo 武漢大學三至九世紀研究所, 281–95. Beijing: Zhongguo Shehuikexue Chubanshe, 2012.

Wang Jiakui王家葵. "Yanzhi jingyi: *Bencao yanyi*" 衍撫經義:《本草衍義》. *Wenshi zhishi* 文史知識 9 (September 2016): 68–74.

Wang Jingbo 王晶波. "Cong dili bowu zaji dao zhiguai chuanqi: *Yiwu zhi* de shengcheng yanbian guocheng ji qi yu gu xiaoshuo de guanxi" 從地理博物雜記到志怪傳奇——《異物志》的生成演變過程及其與古小說的關係. *Xibei shida xuebao (shehuikexue ban)* 西北師大學報 (社會科學版) 34, no. 4 (August 1997): 60–64.

———. "Han Tang jian yiyi Yiwu zhi kaoshu" 漢唐間已佚《異物志》考述. Special issue, *Beijing daxue xuebao* 北京大學學報 37 (December 2000): 178–84.

Wang, Yugen. *Ten Thousand Scrolls: Reading and Writing in the Poetics of Huang Tingjian and the Late Northern Song.* Cambridge, MA: Harvard University Asia Center, 2011.

Watanabe Kōzō 渡邊幸三. "Tō Shinbi no *Kēshi shōrui bikyū honzō* no kētō to sono hanpon" 唐慎微の《經史證類備急本草》の系統とその版本. In *Honzōsho no kenkyū* 本草書の研究, edited by Kyōu Shooku 杏雨書屋, 42–112. Ōsaka: Takeda Kagaku Shinkō Zaidan, 1987.

Wilson, Adrian. "On the History of Disease-Concepts: The Case of Pleurisy." *History of Science* 38 (2000): 271–319.

Wong Cheung-wai 王章偉. "Wenming tuijin zhongde xianshi yu xiangxiang: Songdai Lingnan de wuxi wushu" 文明推進中的現實與想像——宋代嶺南的巫覡巫術. *Xin shixue* 新史學 23, no. 2 (June 2012): 1–55.

Wu Ya-ting 吳雅婷. "Daoting tushuo zhihou: Song Yuan leishu han yishu zhong lüxing shiyong zhishi de tansuo" 道聽途說之後——宋元類書和醫書中旅行實用知識的探索. *Tsinghua xuebao* 清華學報 51, no. 1 (March 2021): 159–98.

Yang, Bin. "The *Zhang* on Chinese Southern Frontiers: Disease Constructions, Environmental Changes, and Imperial Colonization." *Bulletin of the History of Medicine* 84, no. 2 (Summer 2010): 163–92.

Yang, Dolly. "Prescribing 'Guiding and Pulling': The Institutionalisation of Therapeutic Exercise in Sui China (581–618 CE)." PhD diss., University College London, 2018.

Yang Wuquan 楊武泉. "Jiaozhu qianyan" 校注前言. In *Lingwai daida jiaozhu* 嶺外代答校注, 1–16. Beijing: Zhonghua Shuju, 1999.

Ye Fazheng 葉發正. *Shanghan xueshu shi* 傷寒學術史. Wuhan: Huazhong Shifan Daxue Chubanshe, 1995.

Yi Sumei 易素梅. "Songdai de shiren yu yifang: yi *Su Shen neihan liangfang* wei zhongxin de kaocha" 宋代的士人與醫方——以《蘇沈內翰良方》為中心的考察. *Renwen zazhi* 人文雜誌 11 (November 2016): 86–96.

Yu Cailin 余才林. *Tangshi benshi yanjiu* 唐詩本事研究. Shanghai: Shanghai Guji Chubanshe, 2010.

Yu Gengzhe 于賡哲. *Tangdai jibing yiliao shi chutan* 唐代疾病、醫療史初探. Beijing: Zhongguo Shehuikexue Chubanshe, 2011.

Yu Xin 余欣 and Zhong Wumo 鍾無末. "Bowuxue de zhongwan Tang tujing: Yi *Beihu lu* de yanjiu wei zhongxin" 博物學的中晚唐圖景: 以《北戶錄》的研究為中心. *Zhonghua wenshi luncong* 中華文史論叢 118 (June 2015): 313–36, 398–99.

Yu Xinzhong 余新忠. "'Liangyi liangxiang' shuo yuanliu kaolun: jianlun Song zhi Qing yisheng de shehuidiwei" "良醫良相"說源流考論——兼論宋至清醫生的社會地位. *Tianjin shehui kexue* 天津社會科學 4 (July 2011): 120–31.

Zeitlin, Judith. "The Literary Fashioning of Medical Authority: A Study of Sun Yikui's Case Histories." In *Thinking with Cases: Specialist Knowledge in Chinese Cultural History*, edited by Charlotte Furth, Judith Zeitlin, and Ping-chen Hsiung, 169–202. Honolulu: University of Hawai'i Press, 2007.

Zeng Feng 曾鳳. "*Xindiao Sun zhenren qianjin fang* kanke niandai kao" 《新雕孫真人千金方》刊刻年代考. *Beijing zhongyiyao daxue xuebao* 北京中醫藥大學學報 34, no. 5 (May 2011): 306–8.

———. "*Xindiao Sun zhenren qianjin fang* kezhe kao" 《新雕孫真人千金方》刻者考. *Tianjin zhongyiyao* 天津中醫藥 24, no. 6 (December 2007): 492–94.

Zhang, Ellen Cong. "Between Life and Death: Song Travel Writings about *Zhang* 瘴 in Lingnan." *Journal of Song-Yuan Studies* 41 (2011): 191–225.

———. "Of Revelers and Witty Conversationalists: Song (960–1279) *Biji* Writing (Miscellaneous Writing) as Literature of Leisure." *Chinese Historical Review* 23, no. 2 (2016): 130–46.

———. "Things Heard in the Past, Material for Future Use: A Study of Song (960–1279) *Biji* Prefaces." *East Asian Publishing and Society* 6, no. 1 (2016): 22–53.

———. "To Be 'Erudite in Miscellaneous Knowledge': A Study of Song (960–1279) *Biji* Writing." *Asia Major* 25, no. 2 (2012): 43–77.

———. *Transformative Journeys: Travel and Culture in Song China*. Honolulu: University of Hawai'i Press, 2011.

Zhang Haipeng 張海鵬. "Xu Shuwei yizhu zai Nan Song de kanke yu liuchuan" 許叔微醫著在南宋的刊刻與流傳. *Zhonghua yishizazhi* 中華醫史雜誌 45, no. 5 (September 2015): 306–12.

Zhang Hui 張暉. *Songdai biji yanjiu* 宋代筆記研究. Wuchang: Huazhong Shifan Daxue Chubanshe, 1993.

Zhang Kefeng 張軻風. "Cong 'zhang' dao 'zhang': 'Zhang qi' shuo shengcheng de dili kongjian jichu" 從"障"到"瘴": "瘴氣"說生成的地理空間基礎. *Zhongguo lishidili luncong* 中國歷史地理論叢 24, no. 2 (April 2009): 135–43.

Zheng Jinsheng 鄭金生. "*Lü chanyan bencao* jiaozhu houji" 《履巉岩本草》校注後記. In *Nan Song zhenxi bencao sanzhong* 南宋珍稀本草三種, edited by Zheng Jinsheng 鄭金生, 66–77. Beijing: Renmin Weisheng Chubanshe, 2007.

Zhou Yunyi 周雲逸. "*Zhenglei bencao*" yu Songdai xueshu wenhua yanjiu 《證類本草》與宋代學術文化研究. Beijing: Shehuikexue Wenxian Chubanshe, 2017.

Zhu Chongcai 朱崇才. "*Shixian benshi quzi ji* xin kaoding" 《時賢本事曲子集》新考訂. *Wenxian jikan* 文獻季刊 3 (July 2000): 110–23, 160.

Ziporyn, Brook. "Form, Principle, Pattern, or Coherence? Li 理 in Chinese Philosophy." *Philosophy Compass* 3, no. 3 (March 2008): 401–22.

Zou Fuqing 鄒福清. *Tang Wudai biji yanjiu: yi wenren fengqi, wenxue fengqi wei kaoliang zhongdian* 唐五代筆記研究: 以文人風氣、文學風氣為考量重點. Beijing: Zhongguo Shehuikexue Chubanshe, 2013.

Zuo Peng 左鵬. "Han Tang shiqi de *zhang* yu *zhang* yixiang" 漢唐時期的瘴與瘴意象. *Tang yanjiu* 唐研究 8 (December 2002): 257–75.

Zuo, Ya. *Shen Gua's Empiricism*. Cambridge, MA: Harvard University Asia Center, 2018.

Index

Page numbers in *italics* refer to illustrations.

A-B Canon [of Acupuncture] (Jiayi jing), 37–38

abdominal pain, 35

academies and institutes (*guange*), 38–41, 162n81. *See also* Bureau for Editing Medical Texts

Academy of Scholarly Worthies (Jixian Guan), 162n81

Accounts of the Western Regions during the Great Tang (Datang xiyuji), 64

aconite, 116, 117, 120

agarwood, 1

Ai Sheng, *Materia Medica Validated and Classified from the Classics and Histories of the Daguan Reign* (Jingshi zhenglei daguan bencao), 71, 72

air pump, 2

alcoholic drinks, 119–20, 177n65

annotations, 38, 46–47, 102. *See also* *Collected Annotations on the Classic of Materia Medica*

Aoyama Sadao, 167n61

Approaching Correctness (Erya), 56, 64, 168n70

argumentation, 50, 52–53, 65, 70, 71, 72

astragalus (*huangqi*), 97

"attaining knowledge" (*zhizhi*), 54, 165n25

Bai Juyi, 64

Bao Tingbo, edition of *Su's and Shen's Formulas*, 159n34

Basic Questions (Suwen), 53, 66, 98, 99, 100, 125, 178n82

"bedchamber instructions" (*fangzhong*), 12

bee grass (*mifeng cao*), 134

bencao (materia medica), 12. *See also* materia medica

benshi (explanatory historical contexts), 13, 76, 80, 85–89, 102, 140

betel nuts, 119, 121, 127

biji. See notebooks

black ghosts (*wugui*), 60–61, 65

black ram's horns (*guyang jiao*), 44, 48

"blood stasis" (*yuxue*), 44

blue-green wormwood herb (*qinghao*), 128

bodily channels, 21, 125

Bol, Peter, 153n5, 164n17

Book of Songs (Shijing), 83–84

book titles, 18–19, 88, 137, 140, 157n12

botanical treatises, 165n28

Boyanton, Stephen, 172–73n47, 173n67

breast abscesses (*ruyong*), 179n10

Broad Relief (Wangshi boji fang; Wang Gun), 20, 24, 34, 37

"broadness" (*bo*), 58; "broad learning of things" (*bowu*), 59, 167n53

Brown, Miranda, 157n3

Brush Talks from Dream Brook (Mengxi bitan; Shen Kuo): argumentation, 65; "black ghosts" entry, 60–61, 65; "Discussion of Medicinals" (Yaoyi), 64; empirical strategy, 13, 60, 62, 69, 167n58, 167–68n69; epistemological approach, 13, 28–30, 159n45; influence on later notebooks, 42–43; mention of "coherence" (*li*), 65; presentation of knowledge, 29–30; on "rainbow drinking water," 60; as source for Kou's *Elucidating the Meaning*, 64–65; on the "thunder ax," 60

bupleurum (*chaihu*), 115, 126; Major Bupleurum Decoction; 76, 83, 86, 97, 99, 127; Minor Bupleurum Decoction, 117

Bureau for Editing Medical Texts (Jiaozheng Yishuju), 38–39, 42, 101, 161–62n78; edition of *Essential Formulas*, 39–41, 102; edition of *Treatise on Cold Damage*, 101–2; prefaces to medical texts, 39–40

Cai Xiang, *Inventories of Lychee* (Lizhi pu), 64, 65

calendars, 29

"canonical remedies" (*jingfang*), 12

Cao Xiaozhong, 169n99; *Zhenghe Materia Medica* (Zhenghe xinxiu jingshi zhenglei beiyong bencao), 71–72

case narratives: appended to formulas, 41, 83, 85, 86, 102–3, 137, 138; discussion-case-prescription format, 83, 90–91, 103; empirical strategy in, 1–2, 17, 103, 140, 144; in China and Europe, 7, 143; compared to legal cases, 142; function of, 86–87, 103; history of, 5–8, 155n23; intertextual dialogues in, 99–101; of Shen Kuo, 1, 27–28; single-practitioner compilations, 7–8, 17, 155n30; Song and Ming, 139–43, 179n19; physician and nonphysician, 7, 80; structure of, 83, 141–42; of Xu Shuwei, 75, 76–77, 83–84, 86, 90–91, 96–99, 102, 103, 140. *See also* empirical strategy; *Formulary with Explanatory Historical Contexts*; medical case statements genre

censorship, 65

Chanyuan Covenant, 33

Chao Gongwu, *Memoirs of Reading in the Jun Studio* (Junzhai dushu zhi), 25, 126

Chen Baxian (Emperor Wu of Chen), 81, 82

Chen Cangqi, 48; *Collecting the Omissions of Materia Medica* (Bencao shiyi), 47, 52, 57, 60

Chen Cheng, *Expanded Divine Farmer's Materia Medica and Illustrated Materia Medica* (Chongguang buzhu Shennong bencao bing tujing), 46, 71

Chen Hao, 157n8, 164–65n22

Chen Yan, 158n20, 170n104; *Synthesizing Views on Materia Medica in the Baoqing Regime* (Baoqing bencao zhezhong), 136

Chen Yaosou, 110

Chen Yongpei, edition of *Su's and Shen's Formulas*, 159n34

Chen Yuan-peng, 170n7

Chen Zhensun, *Zhizhai's Annotated Catalog* (Zhizhai shulu jieti), 26, 74

Chen Ziming, *Comprehensive Good Medical Formulas for Women* (Furen daquan liangfang), 74, 170n104

Cheng Hao, 54

Cheng Lu, preface to *Stone Mountain Medical Cases*, 142

Cheng Yi, 54

childhood maladies, 89; wet navel, 14, 34

Chinese angelica (*danggui*), 14, 97

Chunyu Yi, 6, 90, 155n23; examination records (*zhenji*), 6, 82, 90

cinnabar pills, 116

cinnamon (*gui*), 177n65

Cinnamon Sea (Guihai yuheng zhi; Fan Chengda), 120, 121, 128, 177n67; entry on *zhang*, 120–21

civil servants. *See* scholar-officials

civil service examinations: and medical practice, 36–37, 77, 78; metropolitan, 79; Song expansion of, 8–9, 36, 123; Xu Shuwei and, 77, 78, 79, 81, 87–88; during Yuan, 170n7

Ciyun Mountain (Zhejiang), 134

classical Chinese medicine, 5, 35, 143–44. *See also* traditional Chinese medicine (TCM)

classified books (*leishu*), 56, 177n67

Classified Cases from Famous Physicians (Mingyi leian), 141

coherence (*li*), 47, 53, 65, 164n17, 165n26, 165n29

coix seeds (*yiyishi*), 105

cold amassment (*hanshan*), 44, 48.

cold damage (*shanghai*) disorders: case narratives of Xu Shuwei, 76–77, 81, 90–91; disputed cases, 96, 103; in the

south, 124–27, 129, 130–31, 178n79, 178n84; treatises, 39, 79–80, 82, 92–96, 99–100, 103, 125, 173n47; and *zhang* disorders, 125–31. *See also One Hundred Questions on Cold Damage*; *Treatise on Cold Damage*; Xu Shuwei

Collected Annotations on the Classic of Materia Medica (Bencaojing jizhu; Tao Hongjing), 46, 47, 49–50, 119–20; entry on fishing cormorants, 49, 51; entry on stonecrops, 52; entry on moles, 52; use of hearsay as persuasion strategy, 49, 52. *See also* Tao Hongjing

Collecting the Omissions (Bencao shiyi; Chen Cangqi), 47, 52, 57, 60

Collection of Effective Formulas (Jiyan fang), 110

Collection of Effective Formulas from Past to Present (Gujin jiyanfang; comp. Xue Jinghui), 19

complexion, 21

Comprehensive Good Medical Formulas for Women (Furen daquan liangfang; Chen Ziming), 74, 170n104

conglomeration diseases (*jijia*), 79

consilium, 143

Construct the Middle Decoction (Jianzhong Tang), 97

Costus Root Pill (Muxiang Wan), 27

Cui Zhiti, *Mr. Cui's Collections of Essential Formulas* (Cuishi zuanyaogfang), 17, 89, 157nn7–8

cultures of reasoning, 154n19

Daguan Materia Medica (Jingshi zhenglei daguan bencao; Ai Sheng), 71, 72

Daizong, Emperor, 69

Daoism, 23, 46, 71, 176n50

Daoist Canons (Daozang jing), 51

INDEX   205

Decoction of Fresh Ginger and Aconite (Shengjiang Fuzi Tang), 116

depletion, 99, 101; colds (*xuhan*), 35

Di Qing, 110–11

diarrhea, 17, 158n27

Directorate of Education (Guozi Jian), 33, 38, 66, 92, 94, 101, 162n92, 168n81

Discerning Cold Damage (Bian shang-han), 92

disease, terms for, 21

Divine Farmer's Classic of Materia Medica (Shennong bencaojing), 38, 46, 50

Divine Pivot (Lingshu), 37, 98

Dong Ji, *Formulary for Travel Houses* (Lüshe beiyao fang), 36, 37

drugs: classification, 69–70; interactions, 22; names, 69; origins, 22; and particularities of patients, 22, 24; preparation, 22; pronunciation and flavor, 53, 164–65n22; testing, 14, 143. *See also* formularies; medical formulas; pharmacological collections

du (poison or toxicity), 112, 176n37. *See also* poison

Du Fu, 61, 64

Du Mu, 64

Duan Chengshi, *Miscellaneous Morsels from Youyang* (Youyang zazu), 58, 64, 87, 167n58

Duan Gonglu, 55–58. See also *Northward-Facing Doors*

dysentery, 97–98

Ebrey, Patricia, 153n5

Edited Materia Medica in the Shaoxing Regime (Shaoxing jiaoding bencao), 74

"effective formulas" (*yanfang*), 18–20, 30, 110, 135; effective-formula strategy, 20, 23

Elucidating the Meaning of Materia Medica (Bencao yanyi; Kou Zong-shi): advantages cited by author, 68–69; argumentation, 50, 52–53, 54, 61, 72; challenges to court-compiled pharmacological texts, 65–66, 68; classification of drugs, 69–70; on "cold amassment" in pregnancy, 44, 48, 74, 170n4; contrasted with Xu Shuwei's *Formulary*, 77; criticism of uncritical acceptance of information, 52; determination of "coherence" (*li*), 50–51, 52, 53–54, 69, 164n17, 165n26; distinguishing features, 47, 54; empirical strategy, 45, 47, 51, 55, 69, 74, 163n1; entry on black ram's horns, 44, 48; entry on fishing cormorants, 48–49, 51, 63; entry on jade spring water, 50–51, 53–54, 69, *73*; entry on moles, 52, 69; entry on "soil made of eastward walls," 52–53, 54, 69; entry on stone honey, 69; entry on water not flowing downward, 69; entry on water passing beneath chrysanthemums, 69; entry on winter ashes, 69; first-person narration, 47, 54, 61; genre-mixing, 49–50; informal style, 47–49, 64, 164n10; information about Kou Zongshi's life, 45; introduction, 45–46; local investigations, 45, 49, 51, 52, 72; medical cases, 44, 48, 49; names of drugs, 69; printings and citation of, 50, 72, *73*, 74; as response to state-commissioned pharmacological encyclopedias, 46–47; on Song medical policies, 66, 67; submission to the court, 65–67, 70, 74; textual sources, 64–65. *See also* Kou Zongshi

empirical strategy: applied to southern disorders, 104–5, 118, 119; approaches

206 INDEX

to, 156n47; in China and Europe, 143; and classical Chinese medicine, 143–44; development of, 2, 13, 132–34, 156n47; and epistemic cultures, 8, 154n19; in Kou Zongshi's *Elucidating the Meaning*, 45, 47, 51, 55, 69, 74; "learned empiricism," 165n30; and local investigations, 55, 56, 57, 165n31; and medical case narratives, 1–2, 5, 17, 103, 140, 144; in *Miscellaneous Morsels*, 167n58; in *Northward-Facing Doors*, 56–57, 58, 59; as persuasion strategy, 2–3, 5, 11, 20, 74, 111, 136, 144; rooted in personal experience, 12, 17, 20, 47; in Shen Kuo's *Brush Talks*, 69, 167n58; in Shen's *Good Formulas*, 20–21; between Song and early Qing, 74, 140; in Southern Song, 134–35; in Sun Simiao's *Essential Formulas*, 17, 156n2; versus textual evidence, 5, 70–71, 136; used by Li Qiu and Wang Fei, 111, 115, 119, 130; in Xue Shuwei's *Formulary*, 103

enchantment disorders, 178n79

ephedra (*mahuang*), 97, 115, 126

epidemics, 38, 91, 161–62n78, 172n43; *zhang* pestilence, 105, 110, 115–16

epistemic autonomy, 10, 12, 13, 87, 132

epistemic cultures, 8–11, 13, 132–33

"epistemic genres" (Pomata), 59

Erya (Approaching correctness), 56, 64, 168n70

Essential Formulas for Urgent Conditions in Lingnan (Lingnan jiyao fang), 109

Essential Formulas Worth a Thousand in Gold, for Emergency Preparedness (Beiji qianjin yaofang; Sun Simiao): and the Bureau for Editing Medical Texs, 38; case records, 18, 89, 90; citation of, 84; criticism by Shen Kuo,

40–41; empirical strategy, 17, 156n2; guide to practicing medicine, 24–25; as *Thousand in Gold*, 22, 23; versions and prefaces, 39–41, 158n25, 162n90. *See also* Sun Simiao

examination records (*zhenji*), 6, 82, 90. *See also* case narratives

experience, concepts of, 153n3. *See also* personal experience

explanatory historical contexts (*benshi*), 13, 76, 80, 85–89, 102, 140

Extensive Accounts of the Reign of Great Peace (Taiping guangji), 60

eye disorders, *16*

"facts" (*shishi*), 13

Fan Chengda, *Treatises of the Supervision and Guardian of the Cinnamon Sea* (Guihai yuheng zhi), 120–21, 128, 177n67

Fan Ka Wai, 157n14, 161n77, 162n78, 169n99, 170n6

Fan Min, 109–10

Fan Ye, biography of Ma Yuan, 105

Fan Yun, 81

fang (methods, formulas, formularies), in formulary titles, 18–19

Fang Chengfeng, 169n89

Fang Qianli, 166n43; *Miscellany of the Wilderness in Which I Was Positioned* (Touhuang zalu), 57

Fang Rui, 167n56

firsthand observation and secondhand experience, 12–13, 26–28, 41–42. *See also* personal experience

Fiscal Commission (Longxing Fu), 72

fishing cormorants (*luci*), 48–49, 51, 61, 63

Five Dynasties and Ten Kingdoms, 109

focal distention (*pi*), 115

foot qi (foot weakness/*jiaoruo*), 17, 112–13, 176n36; *Treatise on Foot Qi in Lingnan* (Lingnan jiaoqi lun; Li Xuan), 109; *zhang* poison foot qi, 112

formularies (*fangshu*): as bibliographic category, 12; case narratives in, 17–18, 75, 76–77, 83–85, 889, 137, 140–41, 142; compiled by Song court, 32, 111, 138–39, 160–61n60, 162–63n92; discussion-case-prescription format, 90; empirical strategy in, 19–20, 134–35; for lay readers, 34, 37, 133; overstatement in, 22; structure and organization, 14–15, 30, 90; Tang, 18, 32, 109, 157n8; titles of, 18–20, 85, 88–89, 137, 140; for travelers, 36; for treating disorders of Lingnan, 107–11, 112–14, 117, 124–25, 127, 129, 130; for treating women, 74. See also *Essential Formulas Worth a Thousand in Gold, for Emergency Preparedness*; *Formulary with Explanatory Historical Contexts*; *Good Formulas*; *Imperial Grace Formulary*; medical case statements genre; medical formulas; pharmacological collections; *Treatise on Cold Damage*; *Treatise on Zhang*

Formulary at the Heart of Medicine (Ishimpō; comp Tamba Yasuyori), 18, 157n10

Formulary for Magnificent Healing and Universal Relief (Shenyi pujiu fang), 32

Formulary for [Ones Staying at] Travel Houses (Lüshe beiyao fang; Dong Ji), 36, 37

Formulary for Saving Life in Lingnan (Lingnan weisheng fang): Jihong's Yuan version, 108; "Ten Talks about the Lingbao Area" (Zhang Jie), 119, 127, 178n88; "Wang Nanrong's Discussion on Remedies and Pulse Diagnosis of Cold and Hot Zhang Disorders," 127–28; Zhang Zhiyuan's version, 107–8, 117, 122, 126. See also *Treatise on Zhang*

Formulary of the Bureau for Benefiting People and Compounding Formulations in an Era of Great Peace (Taiping huimin heji jufang), 139

Formulary That Treats Cold Damage Disorders and Is Bodily Verified (Liao shanghan shen yan fang), 19

Formulary with Explanatory Historical Contexts (Puji benshifang; Xu Shuwei): case narratives, 76–77, 83–84, 86, 90–91, 97, 102, 140; citation of earlier texts, 85, 97, 98, 99, 100; cold damage cases, 76–77, 81, 84, 90–91, 100–101, 103; compared with Liu Xinfu's formulary, 137; compared with *Ninety Discussions*, 80–82; disputed cases, 76, 96–100, 100–101, 173n67; empirical strategy, 103; as first treatise appending medical formulas to cases, 75, 77; inspirations for, 85–86, 102; prefaces, 88–89, 170n1, 171n14; printings, 82; ratio of cases to remedies, 84; targeted reader, 87; title of, 85, 88–89. *See also* Xu Shuwei

Fu, Daiwie, 167n58

Gao Baoheng, 39

Gao Cheng, *Recording the Origins of Things and Affairs* (Shiwu jiyuan), 86

Gao Roune, *Classified and Collected Cold Damage Disorders* (Shanghan zuanlei), 100

Ge Hong, *Kept in One's Sleeve (Formulary*

208 INDEX

Kept in One's Sleeve for Every Emergency; Zhouhou beijifang), 22, 23, 112
Ge Tuan, 115
ginger, 48, 116
Goldschmidt, Asaf, 92, 95–96, 162n78, 171n15, 172n32
Good Formulas (Liangfang; Shen Kuo): audience for, 35, 42; case narratives, 1, 27–28; citation of, 84, 85; on contingent nature of effects, 24, 29, 30; contrasted with Xu Shuwei's *Formulary*, 76; elements of a good formula, 21–24, 25, 41; empirical strategy, 20–21, 43; expanded version, 25–26; "five difficulties" in treating disorders, 21–22, 23, 25; formula for Costus Root Pill, 27; historical significance, 43; narrative form of formulas, 14, 15, *16*; nonsystematic presentation, 29–30; number of individual items, 26, 159n34; preface, 20–24, 25–26, 28, 30, 34, 158n20, 159–60n46, ; sources of formulas, 26–28, 41; and southern disorders, 176n35; title of, 21; "witnessing," 20–21, 22, 23, 25, 26–28, 41–42. See also Shen Kuo; *Su's and Shen's Formulas*
Grand Basis (Taisu), 37
grass *gu*-poisoning, 112, 113
Great Compendium of the Yongle Era (Yongle dadian), 36, 81, 107
Ground Powder of the Seven Preciousnesses (Qibao Cuo San), 116
gu, meaning of, 112
gu-poisoning, 109, 176n39
Guangwu, Emperor, 105
Guangxi, 110–11. See also Lingnan
Guo Tinggui, 135

Han Mao, *Mr. Han's Generalities on Medicine* (Hanshi yitong), 141
Han Qi, 37–38, 39, 161n77
Han Yu, 64
Hanlin Academy, 79, 171n14, 101
Hanson, Marta, 157n12, 177n67
hawksbill turtles (*diamao*), 57
He Yujuan, *Summary of Preserving and Nurturing Life in Guangnan in Four Seasons* (Guangnan sishi sheyang kuozi), 110
healing arts, 22, 29, 42, 158n20
Hinrichs, TJ, 178n79
historicalist-conceptualist approach, 107, 175n12
historiographies, 10, 57, 59, 71, 161n75, 162n80
Historiography Institute (Shi Guan), 162n81
history of knowledge, 8. See also epistemic cultures
history of science and medicine, 4–5, 41–42, 163n96
History of the [Former] Han (Han shu), 12
History of the Later Han (Hou Han shu), 105
History of the South (Nanshi), 81
honey, 69, 134; enema, 76, 97
Hong Mai, *Record of the Listener* (Yijian zhi), 77, 135–36
Hong Zun, *Mr. Hong's Collection of Effective Formulas* (Hongshi jiyan fang), 135
Hu Daojing, 159n32, 159n34
Hu Mian, *Classified Examples of Cold Damage Disorders* (Shanghan leili), 100
Huang Chao's Rebellion, 8
Huang Prefecture (Hubei), 60, 61
Huang Tingjian, 125

Huangfu Mi, 40

Huizong, Emperor: assessment of, 168n79; edict requesting medical formulas, 67–68; imperially brushed edicts, 67–68, 169n89; medical policies, 45, 66–68, 70, 94, 163n1; pharmaceutical collections under, 68, 71–72, 74

Hymes, Robert, 170n7

Illustrated Materia Medica (Bencao tujing), 46, 53, 163n5; classification of drugs, 69–70; criticism and revision, 47, 66, 68, 69–70

Imperial Grace Formulary (Taiping shenghui fang), 14, 32, 66, 93; contrasted with formularies of Li Qiu and Wang Fei, 111–12; on disorders of Lingnan, 112, 113, 114; distributed in Lingnan, 110, 111; prescription strategies, 117; use by lay readers, 34–35

Imperial Library Formulary (Waitai miyao fang, comp. Wang Tao), 18, 38, 40, 157n9, 162n91

Imperial Pharmacy, 138

Imperial Pharmacy's Formulary (Taiyi ju fang), 138–39, 179n14

imperially brushed edicts, 67–68, 169n89

Inner Canon (Huangdi neijing), 98, 105, 138, 173n66

insects, 58

Institute for Collecting and Purchasing Drugs (Shoumai Yaocaisuo), 70

Institute for Extending Literature (Hongwen Guan), 157n9

Institute for the Glorification of Literature (Zhaowen Guan), 40, 162n81

Instructing the Lost (Zhimi fang zhangnüe lun; Wang Fei), 107, 108, 117;

treatments for *zhang* disorders, 104, 111–14, 177n54; use of "heard and saw" (*wenjian*), 118; and Zhou Qufei's *Vicarious Replies*, 121–22. See also Wang Fei

"intermittent fever" (*nüe*), 27, 112, 113, 176nn49–50. See also *zhang* disorders

intertextual dialogues, 99–100, 133

"inventories of things" (*pulu*), 8, 9–10, 55, 64

"investigating things" (*gewu*), 45, 54, 163n1, 165n25

investigations of regional phenomena, 54–57, 63, 65, 72–74, 130, 165n29. See also Lingnan region; travel literature

Jade Spring Temple, 51

jade spring water (*yuquan*), 50–51, 53–54, 69, 164n18; entry from *Newly Compiled and Edited Materia Medica with Illustrations and Commentaries*, 73

Jiahe Powders (Jiahe San), 116

Jianyang, 72, 82

Jiaozhi, 105; Ly Kingdom, 111

Jiayou Materia Medica (*Supplemented and Annotated Divine Farmer's Materia Medica in the Jiayou Regime*/Jiayou buzhu Shennong bencao), 46, 163n5; classification of drugs, 69–70; criticism and revision, 47, 50, 66, 68–69, 70; as textbook, 68

Jihong, *Formulary for Saving Life in Lingnan* (Lingnan weisheng fang), 108. See also *Formulary for Saving Life in Lingnan*

jiji, 101

Jingling bayou (eight companions of the prince of Jingling), 81

Jones, Claire, 156n2

Jurchen Jin, 31, 72, 78–79

Kaibao Materia Medica (Kaibao chong-
ding bencao), 46, 66, 164n18
Kaifeng, 45, 70, 78, 90, 94
Keegan, David, 173n66
Kept in One's Sleeve (Zhouhou beijifang;
Ge Hong), 22, 23, 112
Kou Yue, 50
Kou Zhun, 45
Kou Zongshi: criticism of Tao Hongjing,
52, 63; *Duke Lai's Glorious Loyalty*
(Laigong xunlie), 45; *Elucidating the
Meaning*, 44–45; epistemological
approach, 45; family, 45; official career,
44, 45, 66, 70, 163n3; promotion, 70,
123. See also *Elucidating the Meaning
of Materia Medica*
Kudzu Decoction (Gegen Tang), 101
Kui Prefecture Map Guide (Kuizhou
tujing), 61
Kurz, Johannes, 160n60

Lamb Meat Decoction, 44, 74
lay readers of medical texts, 33–37, 42,
43, 133
"learned empiricism," 165n30
leishu (classified books), 56, 177n67
Leung, Angela, 178n88
li (coherence), 47, 53–54, 65, 164n17,
165n26, 165n29
Li Bai, 64
Li Bo, 62–63
Li Daoyuan, *Commentary on the Classic
of Waterways* (Shuijing zhu), 62–63
Li Jingwei, 160n57
Li Kang, 70
Li Qiu: career and travel, 107, 175n13;
formularies by, 107–8, 111; place of
origin, 108; recovery from *zhang*
pestilence, 104, 115; rejection of existing

formularies for southern disorders,
111–14, 115, 126, 176n35; *Treatise on
Zhang [Miasma] and Intermittent Fe-
ver* (Zhangnüe lun), 104, 107–8, 111–14,
116, 117, 122; use of empirical strategy,
111, 115, 130
Li Shangyin, 51
Li Shuhui, 159n32
Li Xuan, *Treatise on Foot Qi in Lingnan*
(Lingnan jiaoqi lun), 109
Li Zhizhong, 171n14
Li Zhuguo, 38
Liao campaigns, 32–33
Lin Yi, 39–40, 101
Lin'an Prefectural School, 79
Lingnan region: application of cold-damage medicine, 123–25, 178n79; disorders
of, 104–7, 109, 112–13, 114, 122, 174n10;
distribution of medical treatises,
109–11, 130; environment, 118, 126; formularies specific to, 107–11, 112–14, 117,
124–25, 127, 129, 130; healing customs,
104, 109, 134; immigration from north,
109, 126–27; notebook-style writings
on, 56–58, 118–19, 120–23, 130; name
of, 55–56; Song medical campaigns,
109–11, 124, 131; Tang dynasty formularies, 109; as "terroir of flame"
(*yanfang*), 113–14, 176–77n52. See also
Formulary for Saving Life in Lingnan;
Northward-Facing Doors; *Treatise on
Zhang*; *zhang* disorders
"literary technology" (Shapin and Schaffer), 2
literati. See scholar-officials
Liu Ke, 61
Liu Xinfu, *Formulary for Saving Lives
with Factual Evidence* (Huoren
shizheng fang), 137, 141, 142

INDEX 211

Liu Xun, 166n43; *Recording the Extraordinary beyond the Ling Ranges* (Lingbiao luyi), 57, 118–19

Liu Yuanbin, 93

Liu Yuxi, 19; *Passing on Trustworthy Formulas* (Chuanxin fang), 19–20, 23–24, 89, 109, 157n14

Liu Zongyuan, 109

local gazetteers, 63, 119, 130, 177n63

local informants, 74–75

local investigations. *See* investigations of regional phenomena

Lou Yue, 80

Lu Tan, *Correcting Errors in the Easy and Concise Formulary* (Yijian fang jiumiu), 137–38

Lü Wei, 110

Lu Xisheng, 58

Lüchan Rocks (Lüchan yan bencao; Wang Jie), 134

Luo Dajing, *Jade Dew in the Crane Forest* (Helin yulu), 121

"lyrical remarks" (*cihua*) genre, 86

Lyrics with Explanatory Historical Contexts (Shixian benshi quziji; Yang Hui), 85, 86, 87, 102

Ma Yuan, 105

Major Bupleurum Decoction (Da Chaihu Tang), 76, 83, 86, 97, 99, 127

malaria, 106, 174n11, 176n49

manuscript culture, 3. *See also* print culture

Mao Mountain (Jiangsu), 46

map guide (*tujing*) genre, 61, 167n61

Master Tongzhen's Summary of Cold Damage (Tongzhen zi shanghan kuoyao; attrib. Liu Yuanbin), 93

master-disciple transmission, 4, 34, 139–40, 141, 143

materia medica (*bencao*), 12, 32, 46–47, 71–75, 134, 136. See also *Collected Annotations on the Classic of Materia Medica*; *Collecting the Omissions*; *Elucidating the Meaning of Materia Medica*; formularies; *Illustrated Materia Medica*; *Jiayou Materia Medica*; pharmacological collections

Materia Medica Validated and Classified from the Classics and Histories of the Daguan Reign (Jingshi zhenglei daguan bencao; Ai Sheng), 71, 72

medical academies, 31, 67, 168n81, 168n85; Imperial Medical Academy, 66–67, 70; textbook, 68

medical activism. *See* Song medical governance

medical case statements (*yi'an*) genre, 77, 131, 139–43, 154nn20–21; emergence of, 5–8, 80; and European *observationes*, 7; as persuasive strategy, 49. *See also* case narratives

medical education, 4, 33, 38, 66, 68, 69, 93

medical formulas: accompanied by witness statements, 17–23, 26–27, 41, 157n3; accompanying case narratives, 41, 75, 77, 83, 85, 86, 102–3, 137, 138; contingent nature of effects, 24, 29, 30, 158n27; foot weakness, 17; format of, 16, 153n2; Middle English, 156n2; requested by court, 67–68; of scholar-officials, 157n8; sources of, 26–28; use of character *yan* (effective), 17. *See also* drugs; formularies

medical knowledge, transmission of, 4, 20, 86–87, 90, 92; by families and medical lineages, 4, 6, 34, 135, 143; master-disciple, 139–40, 141, 143; public dissemination, 4, 33, 37–38,

43, 78, 133–34; published texts, 4; question-and-answer form, 93–94, 99; self-taught medical learners, 33–34, 37, 78, 117, 143, 161n74

medical marketplace, 138–39

medical texts: attributed to divine figures, 15–17; as authorities, 136, 179n10; as benevolence toward population, 31, 33, 66, 133; categories of, 6–7, 12, 44, 47, 49, 80, 86, 139–43; discussion-case-prescription format, 83, 90–91, 103; edited by scholar-officials, 38–41, 42, 157n8; empirical strategy, 2, 5, 12–13, 134; Han dynasty, 4; lay readers, 33–37, 42, 43, 133; narratives based on personal experience, 1–2, 12–13, 26–28, 47, 58, 87, 154n21; by nonphysicians, 7; and notebook-style writings, 11, 74, 118, 122–23, 130, 133, 177n67; by physician-scholars, 87–88, 138; by physicians, 7, 70–71, 79–80, 136–39; publication media and printing technology, 3–5, 12, 33; question-and-answer form, 93, 99; by self-taught authors, 33–34, 37, 117; Song sponsorship, 3, 4, 32–33, 66–68, 94, 101–2, 133, 160n58, 169n99. *See also* case narratives; empirical strategy; formularies; persuasion strategies

Memoirs of Reading in the Jun Studio (Junzhai dushu zhi; Chao Gongwu), 25, 126

menarche, 102

Meng Qi, *Poems with Explanatory Historical Contexts* (Benshi shi), 85–86, 87, 89, 102, 172n32

Métailié, Georges, 163n1

methods of becoming immortals (*shenxian*), 12

Miao peoples, 112

miasmatic atmosphere (*zhangqi*), 104–5, 106. See also *zhang* (miasma) disorders

middle-period China, 3, 5, 153n5

Minor Bupleurum Decoction (Xiao Chaihu Tang), 117

Minor Construct-the-Middle Decoction (Xiao Jianzhong Tang), 35

Minor Order-the-Qi Decoction (Xiao Chengqi Tang), 97–98

Miscellaneous Morsels from Youyang (Youyang zazu; Duan Chengshi), 58, 64, 87, 167n58

Miscellany of the Wilderness in Which I Was Positioned (Touhuang zalu; Fang Qianli), 57

mist, 118, 119–20, 125

Mo Xiufu, *Records of Wind and Land of Guilin* (Guilin fengtu ji), 57

moles (*yanshu*), 52, 69

Monthly Ordinances (Yueling), 65

morality, 54

mountain dwellers (*shanren*), 47, 60, 61

moxibustion, 104, 128, 135

Mr. Cui's Collections of Essential Formulas (Cuishi zuanyaofang; Cui Zhiti), 17, 89, 157nn7–8

Mr. Seeking Nothing's One Hundred Questions on Cold Damage (Wuqiuzi shanghan baiwen; Zhu Gong), 94

Mr. Wang's Formulary for Broad Relief (Wangshi boji fang; Wang Gun), 20, 24, 34, 37

Mr. Wei's Family Collection of Formulas (Weishi jiacang fang; Wei Xian), 135, 142

Mr. Ye's Collection of Effective Formulas (Yeshi luyan fang; Ye Dalian), 135

musk, 1

INDEX   213

Naitō hypothesis, 155n34
natural history, 167n53
natural-realist approach, 107
neo-Confucianism, 54, 164n17. *See also*
"investigating things"; *li*
New Policies, 31, 61
Newly Compiled and Edited Materia Medica with Illustrations and Commentaries (Xinbian zhenglei tuzhu bencao;
Yu Yanguo Lixian Tang), 72; entry on
jade spring, *73*
*Newly Established Materia Medica in the
Kaibao Regime* (Kaibao xinxiangding
bencao), 32
Newly Revised Materia Medica (Xinxiu
bencao), 46
*Ninety Discussions on Cold Damage
Disorders* (Shanghan jiushi lun; attrib.
Xu Shuwei), 80, 82, 95; authorship of,
80–82, 95–96, 171n20; dating of, 155n30
Nong Zhigao rebellion, 111
north-south axis, 178n88
Northern Dreams (Beimeng suoyan; Sun
Guangxian), 60, 64, 167n56
Northward-Facing Doors (Beihu lu; Duan
Gonglu), 55–59, 87, 166n49; empirical
strategy, 56–57, 58, 59; entry on "*tong
rhinoceros,*" 57; preface by Lu Xisheng,
58–59
notebooks (*biji*), 9–11; accounts of
regional phenomena, 54–55, 57–58,
65, 72–74, 130; empirical strategy in, 8,
13, 60–61; and historiographies, 10, 57,
59; Hong Mai's *Record of the Listener*,
77, 135–36; intertextual dialogue with
medical texts, 133; notebook-style
writings, 74, 87, 118, 122–23, 177n67;
pharmacological knowledge in,
63–64; with prefaces by other authors,

166n47; reliability of, 10–11, 42, 59;
"seeing and hearing" in, 28. See also
Brush Talks from Dream Brook
novels, 58–59
nüe (intermittent fevers), 27, 112, 113,
176nn49–50. See also *zhang* disorders

observationes, 7, 143
Okanishi Tameto, 164n10
One Hundred Questions on Cold Damage
(Shanghan baiwen; Zhu Gong), 67,
93–95
Origins and Symptoms (Zhubing yuanhou
lun), 106, 113, 125
owls (*xiao*), 57

Pang Anshi, 100, 125–26, 178n85; *Discussions on Cold Damage and General
Disorders* (Shanghan zongbing lun),
100, 125
Passing on Trustworthy Formulas (Chuanxin fang; Liu Yuxi), 19–20, 89, 109,
157n14; preface, 19, 23–24
personal experience, 1–2, 12–13, 26–28,
47, 58, 87, 154n21. *See also* empirical
strategy; firsthand observation and
secondhand experience
persuasion strategies, 2–3, 5, 6, 11, 12, 13,
138; asserting "efficacy," 5, 41, 136–37,
140; citing classics as, 5, 138; empirical
evidence as, 2–3, 5, 11, 20, 74, 111, 136,
144; in the formulary genre, 20, 41;
hearsay as, 49, 52; imperial endorsement as, 103; medical cases as, 49,
137, 140, 143; stressing erudition as,
138, 139; textual references as, 46,
70–71, 111, 114, 136; used by physicians,
136–39. *See also* empirical strategy;
personal experience

Peterson, Willard, 164n17

pharmacological collections: criticism of, 61–62, 65–66, 68; European, 163n1; format of entries, 47–49; government-compiled encyclopedias, 32, 46, 68, 71–72, 74, 163n6; under Ming and Qing, 163n6; by physicians, 70–71; textual testimony versus empirical strategies, 70–71. See also *Elucidating the Meaning of Materia Medica*; formularies; materia medica

physicians: from ancient times to Tang, 88; case narratives of, 6–7, 17, 80, 89–91, 141; of Chinese medicine, 7; compared to military strategists, 142; competition for patronage, 77, 90, 140; disputes with household members, 83, 90, 96, 97, 98; education reforms, 66; European, 143; families and lineages, 6, 34, 139–40; formularies by, 18, 24–25; Hippocratic, 42; imperial and lay, 33; in Lingnan, 109, 127; medical texts by, 7, 70–71, 79–80, 136–39; persuasion strategies of, 136–39; scholars as, 67, 87–88, 107, 131, 138; self-taught, 37; Sima Guang on, 22; use of empirical strategy, 17, 136; Xu Shuwei on, 88; during Yuan and Ming, 139–40, 170n7. *See also* Xu Shuwei

"picking-grass-seeds" (*tiao caozi*) technique, 127–28, 129

poetry: cited in medical texts, 51, 61; explanatory historical contexts in, 85–87

poison (*du*), 57, 111, 112, 113–14, 176n37. See also *gu*-poisoning

Pomata, Gianna, "epistemic genres," 59

Powder to Calm the Stomach (Pingwei San), 118

pregnancy, 44, 48

Priceless Qi-Correcting Powder (Buhuan Jin Zhengqi San), 120

print culture, 3–4, 12, 134; woodblock printing, 3, 33, 103. *See also* medical texts

pulse diagnosis, 21, 34, 35, 94, 97, 117–18; texts on, 79, 100, 127, 141

qi: circulated, 29; decoctions for, 97–98, 100, 120; depleted by betel nuts, 127; foot, 17, 109, 112–13, 176n36; hot and cold, 44, 79, 125; normalization of, 17, 104, 116, 120; nutrient, 97; of soil, 52; and *zhang* disorders, 113–14, 115, 120, 121–22, 125, 127

Qian Yi, 89–90

Qingli Reforms, 31

records of exceptional things (*yiwu zhi*), 56–57, 166n39

Records of the [Great] Historian (Shiji; Sima Qian), biography of Chunyu Yi, 6

Records of Wind and Land of Guilin (Guilin fengtu ji; Mo Xiufu), 57

Regulating-Qi Formulary (Tiaoqi fang; attrib. Tanluan), 17–18

reliability of knowledge, 12, 13, 42, 144; in medical texts, 11, 20, 51, 103, 117, 132, 140, 143; notebooks and, 10–11, 42, 59, 87. *See also* scientific knowledge

religious therapies, 113, 160n59

"remedies and techniques" (*fangji*) category, 12, 38

Ren Hong, 38

Renzong, Emperor, 37, 39, 111

Resistant and Withstanding Decoction (Didang Tang), 44

rhinoceros horns, 57

Rose-Storax Pills (Suhexiang Wan), 1

ruyi (scholar-physicians), 67. *See also* physicians: scholars as

Saving Lives (Nanyang huoren shu; Zhu Gong; ed. Zhang Chan), 94–95, 96, 99, 137; imperial endorsement, 103; preface, 100. *See also* Zhu Gong

Sayings of a Female Doctor (Nüyi zayan), 6, 141

scabies, 61

Schaffer, Simon, "literary technology," 2, 153n4

scholar-officials: as authors of formularies, 15, 17, 19–23, 157n8; changes in class composition, 8–9; as editors of medical texts, 38–41, 42, 157n8; investigations of regional phenomena, 45, 55, 63, 72, 165n28; as medical authorities, 37–43, 66–67, 77–78; notebook-style writings, 118, 122–23; Southern Song career paths, 123–24; view of travel, 167n65; views of *zhang* disorders, 127. *See also* civil service examinations; Kou Zongshi; physicians: scholars as; Shen Kuo; Xu Shuwei

scientific knowledge, 2, 29, 143–44, 153n4

"seduction drugs" (*meiyao*), 60

seeing and hearing (*jianwen/wenjian*), 10, 13, 28, 58, 118

sensory perception, 2, 35, 164n22

Sequel to the Classified and Widely Benefiting Formulary with Explanatory Historical Contexts (Leizheng puji benshifang xuji/Benshifang houji), 80

Seven Catalogs (Qilüe), 38, 162n80

shafu (captured by sand), 60

Shao Yong, 142

Shapin, Steven, "literary technology," 2, 153n4

Shen Gua. *See* Shen Kuo

Shen Kuo: *Alternative Orders of Cold Damage Disorders* (Bieci shanghan), 100; and the Bureau for Editing Medical Texts, 40–41, 162n91; case narrative involving, 27; civil service career, 15, 27, 29, 40–41; criteria for good formulas, 40, 41; criticism of court-commissioned formularies, 40–41, 162–63n92; descriptions for lay readers, 37, 133; emphasis on experience, 27–28, 90, 158n17; epistemological approach, 13, 28–30, 42; family and background, 15; influence of, 42–43; lack of medical training, 15; name of, 153n1; scientific and other interests, 29, 160n47; sources of formulas, 26–28; view of profoundness of the universe, 29, 42; on "witnessing," 20–21, 22, 23, 25, 26–28, 41–42, 159–60n46. See also *Brush Talks from Dream Brook*; *Good Formulas*; *Su's and Shen's Formulas*

Shen Pi, 27

Shenzong, Emperor, 89

Shi Kan, 158n27

Shi Zaizhi's Formulary (Shi Zaizhi fang; Shi Kan), 158n27

Sima Guang, 22

Sima Qian, 6

Sivin, Nathan, 158n17

snakes, 61, 112

"soil made of eastward walls" (*dong bitu*), 52–53, 54, 69

soldiers: disorders suffered by, 27, 105, 110, 118; medical resources for, 31, 110–11, 161n77

Song imperial sponsorship of medical

texts, 3, 4, 32–33, 66–68, 94, 101–2, 133, 160n58, 169n99

Song medical governance, 31–32, 43, 66–68, 78, 140, 160n57, 168n81, 170n6; campaigns in Lingnan, 109–11, 124, 131

southern China, 55–56. *See also* Lingnan region

spirit mediums (*wu*), 109, 138

State Affairs, Department of (Shangshu Sheng), 70

Stone Bell Mountain, 62–63

stone honey, 69

Stone Mountain Medical Cases (Shishan yi'an), 6, 141; preface by Cheng Lu, 142

stonecrops (*jingtian*), 52

Straightforward Rhymes of Medicines for and Syndromes of Children (Xiaoer yaozheng zhijue), 89–90, 102–3

Su Mai, 62

Su Shi, 61, 125, 178n85; "Account of a Trip to the Stone Bell Mountain" (Shizhongshan ji), 62–63; writings about medicine, 25, 159n32, 177n65. *See also* *Su's and Shen's Formulas*

Su Song, 39–40

Sui Dynasty History (Sui shu), imperial bibliography, 19

Suichu Hall Catalog (Suichu tang shumu; You Mao), 26

Sun Guangxian, 60; *Trifling Talks from Northern Dreams* (Beimeng suoyan), 60, 64, 167n56

Sun Qi, 39

Sun Simiao, 17, 18, 88, 177n65; *Supplement to Formulas Worth a Thousand in Gold*, 92. *See also* *Essential Formulas Worth a Thousand in Gold, for Emergency Preparedness*

Sun Zhao, *Rhymed Instructions on the Pulse Patterns of Cold Damage Disorders* (Shanghan maijue), 100

Sun Zhining, 137–38

sunlight, 52–53, 56

Su's and Shen's Formulas (Su Shen neihan liangfang), 25–26, 159n32; dosages of ingredients, 162n92; editions of, 159n34; sources of formulas, 26–27, 28. See also *Good Formulas*

sweating 76, 99, 101, 117; treatment by, 97, 126

Taizong, Emperor, 32, 160–61n60

Taizu, Emperor, 32

tales (*xiaoshuo*), 10, 58–59

Tamba Yasuyori, *Formulary at the Heart of Medicine* (Ishimpō), 18, 157n10

Tang Shenwei: *Materia Medica Validated and Classified from the Classics and Histories for Emergency Preparedness* (Jingshi zhenglei beiji bencao), 70–71, 169n98

Tanluan, 17–18

Tao Hongjing (Yinju), 46, 48–49, 52, 63, 177n6. See also *Collected Annotations on the Classic of Materia Medica*

tong rhinoceros (*tongxi*), 57

traditional Chinese medicine (TCM), 32, 98, 144. *See also* classical Chinese medicine

Transcendent Canon (Xianjing), *Thirty-Six Methods of Water*, 164n18

travel literature, 8, 9, 10, 55; accounts of regional phenomena, 65, 72–74; Buddhist, 64; empirical strategy in, 62–63

Treatise on Cold Damage (Shanghan lun; Zhang Ji), 35, 39, 66, 95; canonization of, 91–93, 95–96, 102, 103, 111, 173n47; citation of, 35, 97, 98, 99–100, 101, 138;

INDEX   *217*

Treatise on Cold Damage (continued)
court-commissioned version, 101–2; lack of treatments for southern disorders, 126; and *One Hundred Questions*, 67, 93–94; origin story, 91–92; preface to the edited version, 39, 40; and Xu Shuwei's cold damage treatises, 95

Treatise on Origins and Symptoms of All Disorders (Zhubing yuanhou lun), 106, 113, 125

Treatise on Zhang (Zhangnüe lun; Li Qiu), 104, 111–14; and *Formulary for Saving Life in Lingnan*, 107–8; remedies, 116; Wang Fei's view of, 117; and Zhang Zhiyuan's treatise, 107–8, 117, 122, 126. See also *Formulary for Saving Life in Lingnan*

turtle shell (*biejia*), 115

Unschuld, Paul, 163n1, 173n66

Validated and Classified (Jingshi zhenglei beiji bencao; Tang Shenwei), 70–71, 169n98

Vicarious Replies from beyond the Ling Ranges (Lingwai daida; Zhou Qufei), 121–23, 129–30, 177n67

Wang Fangqing, *Formulary for Lingnan* (Lingnan fang), 109

Wang Fei: *Formulary for Instructing the Lost* (Zhimi fang zhangnüe lun), 104, 107, 108, 111–14, 117–18, 121–22, 177n54; rejection of existing formularies, 111–14, 127; routine for maintaining health, 118, 120; study of medicine, 117; use of empirical strategy, 117, 130; view of muteness-causing *zhang*, 127, 129; as Wang Nanrong, 127–29

Wang Gun, *Mr. Wang's Formulary for Broad Relief* (Wangshi boji fang), 20, 24, 34, 37

Wang Jie, *Materia Medica on Lüchan Rocks* (Lüchan yan bencao), 134

Wang Jingbo, 166n39

Wang Jizhi, 115

Wang Shi, 100

Wang Tao, *Imperial Library Formulary* (Waitai miyao fang), 18, 38, 40, 157n9, 162n91

Wang Zijin, 107

way of medicine, 88

Wei He, 56

Wei Xian, *Mr. Wei's Family Collection of Formulas* (Weishi jiacang fang), 135, 142

Wendi, 106

Western medicine, 7, 143

wet navel malady, 14, 34

White Tiger Decoction (Baihu Tang), 101, 115, 126

wind, 29, 61, 101, 113, 126, 127

"witnessing" (*mudu*). *See* Shen Kuo

woodblock printing, 3, 33, 103

wormwood (*ai*), 53; blue-green wormwood herb (*qinghao*), 128

Wu, Emperor, of Chen (Chen Baxian), 81, 82

Wu, Emperor, of Liang (Xiao Yan), 81, 82

Wu Kun, *Language of Pulse Patterns* (Maiyu), 141

Xiao Yan (Emperor Wu of Liang), 81, 82

Xie Fugu, 101

Xu Shuwei: and the civil service examinations, 77, 78, 79, 81, 87–88; cold damage treatises, 79–80, 82, 95–96; family, 77, 88, 170n1; life and works,

77–82; official career, 79, 171nn14–15; practice of medicine, 77, 79, 87. *See also Formulary with Explanatory Historical Contexts*; *Ninety Discussions on Cold Damage Disorders*

xue (blood), 97, 173n63; blood stasis, 44

Xue Jinghui, *Collection of Effective Formulas from Past to Present* (Gujin jiyanfang), 19

yan (verify/effective), 17, 18, 25. *See also* "effective formulas"

Yan Jizhong, 89–90

Yan Shigu, 56

yang brightness (*yangming*), 76, 99, 128

Yang Hui (Yuansu), *Lyrics with Explanatory Historical Contexts* (Shixian benshi quziji), 85, 86, 87, 102

Yang Shiying, 136–37

Yang Zhong, 105

Yangdi, 106

Yangzi River transport network, 78

Ye Dalian, *Mr. Ye's Collection of Effective Formulas* (Yeshi luyan fang), 135

Ye Linzhi, 142

Yellow Dragon Decoction Formula, 162n91

Yellow Emperor medical tradition, 53, 98, 99, 173n66. *See also Basic Questions*; *Yellow Emperor's Inner Canon*

Yellow Emperor's Inner Canon (Huangdi neijing), 98, 105, 138, 173n66

yi (medicine), 12, 156n45

Yi Sumei, 159n33, 162–63n92

yi'an. See medical case statements genre

Yizhen Gazetteer (Yizhen zhi), 79

You Mao, *Suichu Hall Catalog* (Suichu tang shumu), 26

Yu Xin, 165n31

Yu Yanguo Lixian Tang, *Newly Compiled and Edited Materia Medica with Illustrations and Commentaries* (Xinbian zhenglei tuzhu bencao), 72, 73

Yue Fei, 171n15

Zeng Xie, 171n14

Zhang, Emperor, of Han, 105

Zhang Chan, 94, 100. *See also Saving Lives*

Zhang Ding, 115

zhang (miasma) disorders: alcohol as prevention, 119–20, 177n65; application of cold-damage medicine, 125–31; associated with environment, 104, 105–6, 113, 114, 120–21; attributed to poisons, 113–14; character *zhang*, 105, 174n7; cold *zhang* and hot *zhang*, 114, 122, 127–28, 129; misdiagnosis, 115, 178n88; mountain *zhang*–intermittent fever (*shan zhangnüe*), 112, 113; muteness-causing *zhang* (*yazhang*), 122, 127, 129; in notebook-style writings, 119–23; pulse diagnosis, 117; qi and, 113–14, 115, 120, 121–22, 125, 127; translation of, 106, 174n11, 176n49; treatises, 106, 107–8, 119, 122; treatments, 104, 114, 116, 120–21, 127, 128–29, 177n65; 178n88; *zhang* epidemics, 105, 110, 115–16. *See also Formulary for Saving Life in Lingnan*; *Instructing the Lost*; *Treatise on Zhang*

Zhang Haipeng, 171n14

Zhang Ji (Zhongjing), 48, 91–92, 172n44; *Treatise on Cold Damage and Miscellaneous Disorders* (Shanghan zabing lun), 91–92, 93, 172n43; *Treatise on Cold Damage Disorders* (Shanghan lun), 35, 39, 90–91; treatises attributed

INDEX *219*

Zhang Ji (*continued*)
to, 92–93, 173n47; untransmitted treatments, 76. See also *Treatise on Cold Damage*

Zhang Jie, "Ten Talks about the Lingbiao Area" (*Lingbiao shishuo*), 119, 127, 178n88

Zhang Kefeng, 174n7

Zhang Lei, *Mingdao's Miscellany* (Mingdao zazhi), 61–62

Zhang Yu, 79

Zhang Zhiyuan, treatise on *zhang*, 107–8, 117, 122, 126. See also *Formulary for Saving Life in Lingnan*

Zhang Zhongjing. *See* Zhang Ji

Zhang Zhongjing's Lamb Meat Decoction, 44, 48

Zhanglun, 174n1. See also *Treatise on Zhang*

Zhao Xuemin, *Supplement to Systematic Materia Medica* (Bencao gangmu shiyi), 75

Zhen Prefecture (Jiangsu), 78–79, 82

Zheng Jingxiu, *Treatise and Formulary for Preserving Life in Guangnan in Four Seasons* (Guangnan sishi shesheng fang lun), 109, 110

Zhenghe Materia Medica (Zhenghe xinxiu jingshi zhenglei beiyong bencao; Cao Xiaozhong), 71–72, 169n99

Zhizhai's Annotated Catalog (Zhizhai shulu jieti; Chen Zhensun), 26, 74

Zhong Wumou, 165n31

Zhou Qufei, 121; *Vicarious Replies from beyond the Ling Ranges* (Lingwai daida), 121–23, 129–30, 177n67

Zhu Gong: cited by Xu Shuwei, 96, 100; court appointment, 94, 99; *Mr. Seeking Nothing's One Hundred Questions on Cold Damage* (Wuqiuzi shanghan baiwen), 94; *One Hundred Questions on Cold Damage* (Shanghan baiwen), 67, 93–95; *Saving Lives* (Nanyang huoren shu), 94–95, 96, 99, 100, 103, 137

Zou Fuqing, 166n47

Zuo, Ya, 156n47, 167–68n69

Index **221**

222 *Index*

Milton Keynes UK
Ingram Content Group UK Ltd.
UKHW010302020524
442015UK00003B/44